Cardiovascular and Thoracic Anaesthesia

Anaesthesia in a Nutshell

Commissioning Editor: Michael Parkinson
Project Development Manager: Clive Hewat
Project Manager: Frances Affleck
Designer: George Ajayi

Cardiovascular and Thoracic Anaesthesia

Anaesthesia in a Nutshell

John Gothard MBBS FRCA
Consultant Anaesthetist
Royal Brompton Hospital
London, UK

Andrea Kelleher MBBS FRCA
Consultant Anaesthetist
Royal Brompton Hospital
London, UK

Elizabeth Haxby MBBS FRCA
Consultant Anaesthetist
Royal Brompton Hospital
London, UK

Series Editors: **Neville Robinson and George Hall**

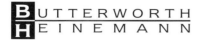

Edinburgh London New York Oxford Philadelphia St Louis Sydney Toronto 2003

BUTTERWORTH-HEINEMANN
An imprint of Elsevier Science Limited
© 2003, Elsevier Science Limited. All rights reserved.

First published 2003

ISBN 0750653558

British Library Cataloguing in Publication Data
A catalogue record for this book is available from the British Library

Library of Congress Cataloging in Publication Data
A catalog record for this book is available from the Library of Congress

Notice
Medical knowledge is constantly changing. Standard safety precautions must be followed, but as new research and clinical experience broaden our knowledge, changes in treatment and drug therapy may become necessary or appropriate. Readers are advised to check the most current product information provided by the manufacturer of each drug to be administered to verify the recommended dose, the method and duration of administration, and contraindications. It is the responsibility of the practitioner, relying on experience and knowledge of the patient, to determine dosages and the best treatment for each individual patient. Neither the Publisher nor the authors assumes any liability for any injury and/or damage to persons or property arising from this publication.

The Publisher

 ELSEVIER SCIENCE

your source for books, journals and multimedia in the health sciences

www.elsevierhealth.com

The publisher's policy is to use paper manufactured from sustainable forests

Printed in China

Contents

Series preface

Specialist registrars and senior house officers in anaesthesia are now trained by the use of modular educational programmes. In these short periods of intense training the anaesthetist must acquire a fundamental understanding of each anaesthetic speciality. To meet these needs, the trainee requires a concise, pocket-sized book that contains the core knowledge of each subject.

The aims of these 'nutshell' guides are two-fold: first, to provide trainees with the fundamental information necessary for the understanding and safe practice of anaesthesia in each speciality; and secondly, to cover all the key areas of the fellowship examination of the Royal College of Anaesthetists and so act as revision guides for trainees.

P. N. Robinson
G. M. Hall

Preface

This new volume in the *Anaesthesia in a Nutshell* series is intended primarily for anaesthetists in training. Nurses, physiotherapists, anaesthetic technicians and surgical trainees involved in the perioperative care of patients with cardiovascular and thoracic disease should also find the book useful.

We have attempted to cover the three topics of cardiac, vascular and thoracic anaesthesia in a succinct and straightforward manner to comply with the aims of the *Nutshell* series. At the same time we have provided sufficient up-to-date information for those anaesthetists taking the Final FRCA Examination. It is also intended that the book will provide a practical guide and overview for those anaesthetists encountering cardiovascular and thoracic anaesthesia for the first time.

We are grateful to Professor George Hall for his skilful editing of our original manuscript and to the publishers for their support. As always we also thank our families for their unfailing support during a project of this nature.

John Gothard
Andrea Kelleher
Elizabeth Haxby

Preoperative assessment for cardiac surgery

A thorough preoperative assessment facilitates an informed estimate of perioperative risk, identifies patients requiring additional investigations and medical intervention and allows the anaesthetist to plan perioperative care. The assessment should be undertaken by the anaesthetist who will be involved in the intraoperative care of the patient. This usually takes place the night before surgery, although many patients are now seen in preoperative assessment clinics several days before admission.

The results of all routine investigations should be available, including blood tests and cardiological investigations. Details of the history and examination may require more attention, particularly those relating to the airway and presence of comorbid disease. Patients admitted as emergencies may not have had a routine 'work-up' and further investigations may be indicated, such as lung function tests in patients with chronic airways disease.

The preoperative visit allows the patient to gain information about the anaesthetic. Some units provide leaflets and videos before admission but a direct discussion allays anxiety. Details about fasting and premedication should be clearly explained, with a description of what will happen in the anaesthetic room. This should include the application of monitoring and siting of cannulae under local anaesthetic. It is prudent to discuss the possibility of blood transfusion and techniques such as cell-salvage. We include a section on the preoperative assessment form for the anaesthetist to indicate what has been discussed.

Assessment of risk

Almost one-third of the population dies from coronary artery disease, and cardiac surgery offers the potential for considerable benefit to a large number of people. The UK Cardiac Surgical Register collects annual cardiac surgical activity and mortality data from each NHS cardiothoracic surgical unit. Over 38 000 (70% for coronary disease) cardiac operations were carried out in the year 1999–2000 with an

---

Table 1.1   Factors associated with increased operative mortality during CABG

Surgery

Increased age	Female gender
Urgent or emergency surgery	Low ejection fraction
Left mainstem coronary disease	Repeat surgery
Diabetes	Renal impairment
Hypertension	Peripheral vascular disease

---

overall mortality of 3.9%. For isolated coronary artery bypass grafting (CABG), the average mortality is 2.2% in the UK. Factors associated with increased operative mortality are shown in Table 1.1.

CABG is performed for the relief of angina and the prolongation of life. The accepted scoring system for angina is the Canadian Cardiovascular Society (CCS) grading system (Table 1.2) (higher scores indicate more severe angina.) Approximately 20% of patients presenting for CABG have severe angina (CCS4) with an overall mortality of 4.2%. Breathlessness is graded according to the New York Heart Association Classification (NYHA) (Table 1.3). Patients in NYHA 4 have a 6.6% mortality following CABG surgery.

Table 1.2   Canadian Cardiovascular Society classification of effort angina

Class I	Ordinary physical activity does not cause angina. Angina occurs with strenuous or rapid or prolonged exertion at work or recreation
Class II	Slight limitation of ordinary activity. Angina occurs with walking or climbing stairs rapidly, walking uphill, walking, or stair climbing after meals, or in the cold, or in wind, or under emotional stress, or only during the few hours after awakening. Angina occurs when walking more than two blocks on the level or climbing more than one flight of stairs at a normal pace and in normal conditions
Class III	Marked limitation of ordinary physical activity. Angina occurs with walking one to two blocks on the level and climbing one flight of stairs in normal conditions at a normal pace
Class IV	Inability to carry on any physical activity without discomfort — angina may be present at rest

Table 1.3   New York Heart Association Functional Classification

Class I	Patients with cardiac disease but without resulting limitations of physical activity. Ordinary physical activity does not cause undue fatigue, palpitations, dyspnoea or anginal pain
Class II	Patients with cardiac disease resulting in slight limitation of physical activity. They are comfortable at rest. Ordinary physical activity results in fatigue palpitations, dyspnoea or anginal pain
Class III	Patients with cardiac disease resulting in marked limitation of physical activity. They are comfortable at rest. Less than ordinary physical activity causes fatigue, palpitations, dyspnoea or anginal pain
Class IV	Patients with cardiac disease resulting in inability to carry on any physical activity without discomfort. Symptoms of cardiac insufficiency or of the anginal syndrome may be present even at rest. If any physical activity is undertaken discomfort is increased

A number of risk stratification systems for cardiac surgery have evolved, including logistic regression and Bayes modelling techniques. These range from simple additive systems (Parsonnet) to highly complex statistical algorithms.

The Parsonnet scoring system was developed in North America in 1989. A score is calculated before the operation and a higher score indicates increased risk. Although most of the variables in the Parsonnet system remain pertinent, their impact on mortality has changed over the last 10 years. More recently, a Pan-European scoring system (EURO SCORE) (Table 1.4) has been developed with slightly different risk factors and weightings making allowances for advances in surgical practice and a different patient population. It is a weighted, additive score and the weights add up to approximate percentage predicted mortality. Most patients have a score between 0 and 3, which approximates to a risk of death in the range 0% to 3%. This scoring system, when applied to over 16 000 patients from the UK cardiac surgical database, was found to give a better estimate of operative mortality than Parsonnet.

Bayesian analyses have also been used in predicting risk. The Bayesian table is a simple way of building risk stratification systems from a database. Based on tables relating outcome to single risk factors, the probability of an adverse outcome can be estimated for a patient with any combination of risk factors. Comparison of currently available

Table 1.4 European System for Cardiac Operative Risk evaluation Score (EuroSCORE). (Adapted from Nashef et al. 1999)

Factor	Definition	Score
Age	Per 5 years or part thereof	1
Gender	Female	1
Chronic pulmonary disease	Long-term use of bronchodilators or steroids for lung disease	1
Extracardiac arteriopathy	Any one or more of the following: claudication carotid occlusion or > 50% stenosis, previous or planned surgery on the abdominal aorta, limb arteries or carotids	2
Neurological dysfunction	Disease severely affecting ambulation or day-to-day functioning	2
Previous cardiac surgery	Previous surgery requiring opening of the pericardium	3
Serum creatinine	> 200 mmol/l preoperatively	2
Active endocarditis	Patient still under antibiotic treatment for endocarditis at the time of surgery	3
Critical preoperative state	Ventilation before arrival in the anaesthetic room, preoperative inotropic support, intra-aortic balloon pump, or preoperative acute renal failure	3
Unstable angina	Angina requiring intravenous nitrates until arrival in anaesthetic room	2
Left ventricular dysfunction	Moderate (ejection fraction 30% to 50%) Poor ejection fraction < 30%	1 3
Recent myocardial infarction	< 90 days	2
Pulmonary hypertension	Systolic pulmonary artery pressure > 60 mmHg	2
Emergency	Carried out on referral before next working day	2
Other than isolated coronary artery bypass surgery	Major cardiac operation other than or in addition to coronary artery bypass surgery	2
Surgery on thoracic aorta	Ascending, arch or descending aorta	3
Postinfarction septal rupture		4

Table 1.5   UK Cardiac Surgical Register Summary Data 1999–2000

Procedure	Number	% Mortality
Isolated valve surgery	5393	5.5
Isolated coronary artery surgery	24 728	2.2
Combined coronary and valve surgery	2641	7.8
Other operations for ischaemic heart disease	462	17.2
Congenital	3876	4.2
Miscellaneous	1409	15.8
Total	38 509	3.9

scoring systems indicates that Parsonnet no longer reflects risk accurately; the Euroscore is an improvement but Bayes scores, trained on the most recent UK cardiac surgical data available, provide an even more accurate prediction (Table 1.5.)

Recently, the Cardiac Anaesthesia Risk Evaluation Score (CARE) was found to be a clinically useful predictor of mortality and morbidity after cardiac surgery. It is a simple classification based on clinical judgement and three clinical variables: (1) comorbid conditions categorized as controlled or uncontrolled, (2) surgical complexity and (3) urgency of surgery. The CARE score performs well against Parsonnet and other multifactorial risk indices.

General anaesthetic assessment

Whilst the patient may have been extensively investigated, information of specific interest to the anaesthetist may not be documented. Airway assessment is important; patients with rheumatoid arthritis or ankylosing spondylitis often present for valve surgery and may require fibreoptic intubation. A history of smoking is relevant because it is associated with impaired lung function and also peripheral vascular disease. The presence of the latter has important implications, including the possibility of carotid disease requiring surgery, aortic atheroma, which may make application of the aortic cross clamp hazardous, and renal artery stenosis and iliofemoral disease, which can make femoral artery cannulation and passage of an intra-aortic balloon pump difficult. A neurological examination should be carried out to document any pre-existing deficits. Routine questioning about allergies, previous anaesthetics and drug history are vital because a number of medications such as aspirin have implications for surgery. Patients with pacemakers should have these checked before surgery.

The results of all preoperative investigations should be available including the echocardiography report and angiography results, particularly ejection fraction and left ventricular end-diastolic pressure. Lung function tests and findings on chest radiograph are useful as a baseline and arterial blood gases may be indicated in those with impaired lung function.

The increasing use of normothermia or moderate hypothermia during cardiopulmonary bypass, and off-pump surgery, has meant that it is possible for selected patients undergoing routine surgery to be extubated early in the postoperative period. An attempt may be made to identify such patients preoperatively but the selection criteria vary between units. However, intraoperative events influence outcome as much as preoperative status and patients identified as suitable for a 'fast-track' approach do not always remain on this pathway. The anaesthetic approach to such patients is discussed further in Chapter 2.

Preoperative tests

A number of routine and specialised tests are undertaken before surgery (Table 1.6).

Full blood count

Anaemia should be investigate before surgery and treated appropriately. Significant haemodilution occurs during cardiopulmonary bypass and may require blood transfusion or haemofiltration to maintain adequate oxygen carriage if preoperative haemoglobin is less than 10 g/dl. Anaemia of chronic disease and that associated with haemoglobinopathies can be treated with blood transfusion. Patients with chronic renal failure are often anaemic but should not have their haemoglobin levels elevated rapidly by transfusion because this may precipitate cardiac failure. Anaemia resulting from gastrointestinal pathology is significant as bleeding may be exacerbated by full heparinisation required for cardiopulmonary bypass. Postoperative gastrointestinal-haemorrhage requiring surgery carries a high mortality. It is essential to optimize haemoglobin levels preoperatively with iron supplements and other agents such as erythropoetin. Platelet function may be abnormal due to aspirin therapy and further damage occurs during cardiopulmonary bypass. A low platelet count should be investigated and treated, if necessary, with platelet transfusions.

Coagulation studies

Drug therapy and abnormal liver function are the main causes of coagulopathy preoperatively. Aspirin and dipyridamole both inhibit platelet

Table 1.6 Preoperative laboratory investigations

Routine tests	Tests as indicated
Full blood count	Liver function
Coagulation profile	Lipid profile
Urea and electrolytes	Thyroid function
Serum creatinine	Hepatitis status
Serum glucose	MRSA status
Group and save/crossmatch (as per unit policy)	

activity and non-steroidal anti-inflammatory drugs (NSAIDS) have a similar effect. Patients with unstable angina may be given intravenous or subcutaneous heparin and, if they have recently undergone angioplasty or stent insertion, may have received thrombolytic agents such as streptokinase or platelet GPIIb-IIIa inhibiting agents.

Abnormal liver function increases the risk associated with surgery, and poor perfusion during surgery may impair liver function further reducing clotting factor production. Abnormal clotting of unknown aetiology requires investigation before surgery. Known clotting defects should be treated appropriately with fresh frozen plasma, platelets, antifibrinolytics, vitamin K and specific factor concentrates.

Urea creatinine and electrolytes
Patients with pre-existing renal impairment are at high risk of developing postoperative renal failure, which has a high mortality. The causes are often multifactorial but include diabetes, hypertension and renal artery stenosis. The latter should be treated before surgery is undertaken. Creatinine clearance is a useful measurement and indicates the extent of renal impairment more reliably than serum creatinine. Urine output and renal function should be closely monitored during the perioperative period and, although many different techniques have been used to prevent the onset of renal failure, none have been found to be effective. At risk patients should be kept well hydrated and all nephrotoxic drugs avoided.

Patients with chronic renal failure commonly present for coronary artery surgery. Close liaison with renal physicians about dialysis, both pre- and postoperatively, is essential. Abnormalities of serum sodium, potassium and magnesium are common in these patients because of chronic diuretic therapy and beta blockade. In most patients, treatment is unnecessary and correction can be undertaken intraoperatively, particularly for potassium and magnesium.

Liver function tests
Impaired liver function usually results from right heart failure or excessive alcohol intake. Occasionally, patients present with more unusual forms of liver disease. Clotting abnormalities and altered drug metabolism are the main problems associated with liver impairment.

Blood glucose
Diabetes is very common in patients presenting for cardiac surgery and, occasionally, it is discovered during preparation for surgery. Many patients are adequately controlled with dietary restriction and oral hypoglycaemics, but an increasing number of diabetics are maintained on insulin. Diabetic patients can have significant end-organ damage, particularly in the kidney. Insulin regimens in the perioperative period vary between hospitals but careful control of blood sugar is important.

Cardiological investigations
Chest X-ray
Although the cost-effectiveness of routine chest radiography has been questioned, it is probably justified before cardiac surgery. Postero–anterior films are taken routinely and show the shape and size of the heart, great vessels, lung vasculature, presence of valve calcification and pleural or pericardial effusions. Lateral films may be useful in patients undergoing reoperation to demonstrate the proximity of the heart and great vessels to the back of the sternum; most patients have a normal chest radiograph, which acts as a useful baseline in the postoperative period. Isolated cardiomegaly in the absence of congenital or valvular heart disease implies a degree of ventricular dysfunction.

Electrocardiogram
Abnormalities of the pre-operative 12-lead electrocardiogram (ECG) are common, usually ST segment changes, but also Q waves, rhythm disturbances and conduction abnormalities. The preoperative ECG should be performed 24–48 h before surgery, particularly in patients with unstable angina because many infarcts are silent and new changes are significant. A normal ECG does not exclude ischaemia and acts a baseline postoperatively.

Exercise tolerance test

The exercise tolerance test (ETT) is often the initial diagnostic test performed in patients with stable angina with a borderline or normal resting ECG. It is undertaken to assess functional capacity and a 12-lead ECG is recorded before, during and after graded exercise on a treadmill or bicycle ergometer. Many exercise protocols exist and the primary goal is to increase the workload of the heart to elicit maximal oxygen consumption. There is an approximately linear increase in heart rate as myocardial oxygen consumption rises during exercise. The duration of exercise and heart rate at the onset of ischaemic pain or ECG changes are reproducible indices of the severity of myocardial ischaemia.

The ETT can provide information in three areas; ischaemia, ventricular dysfunction and arrhythmias. The most widely accepted ECG criterion for ischaemia is ST segment depression of at least 1 mm at 0.08 s after the end of the QRS complex. An ETT is considered strongly positive of left mainstem or three-vessel coronary artery disease when the systolic blood pressure drops by 10 mmHg or more, more than five leads show positive ST segment changes, and ischaemic changes occur within 3 min and take more than 9 min to resolve. The test is stopped if the patient experiences symptoms, develops ST segments changes of greater than 2 mm, a fall in blood pressure of greater than 15 mmHg or ventricular arrhythmias. Ischaemia or arrhythmias occurring at rest after exercise are worrying. Contraindications and limitations to the ETT are shown in Table 1.7. From the anaesthetic viewpoint, a positive ETT indicates a higher risk patient.

Perfusion imaging

The ETT can be enhanced by injecting intravenous thallium-201 or the newer agent technetium-99 during peak exercise and measuring

Table 1.7 Contraindications and limitations to exercise tolerance tests

Contraindications to ETT	Limitations
Aortic stenosis	Peripheral vascular disease may limit exercise capacity
Acute myocardial infarction within 7 days	Electrocardiogram abnormalities may preclude analysis (e.g. left bundle branch block)
Pulmonary hypertension	Beta blockers limit peak heart rate
Unstable angina	

regional myocardial perfusion with a gamma camera. Imaging is performed within 30 min of exercise and 2–4 h later. Hypoperfused areas initially appear as image defects, which may recover after a period of rest (reversible defects). This may indicate that revascularization is appropriate. Persistent defects indicate non-viable myocardium.

Patients who are unable to exercise may be 'stressed' by pharmacological means using dypiridamole, adenosine or dobutamine. These vasodilators cause maximal dilatation of coronary arteries. Vessels with fixed stenoses do not dilate, resulting in preferential distribution of blood flow, and hence thallium, away from the areas supplied by stenotic vessels towards the normally supplied areas. This is identified as a perfusion defect on the scan. Dobutamine, at a high dose, increases blood pressure and heart rate and perfusion imaging has been shown to have high specificity and sensitivity for detecting ischaemic heart disease.

Contraindications to myocardial perfusion imaging in conjuction with dypiridamole, adenosine or dobutamine

- Unstable angina.
- Acute myocardial infarction within 48 h.
- Bronchospasm.
- Allergy to dypiridamole or thallium.

Echocardiography

Advances in echocardiography have increased its usefulness before cardiac surgery and it is now undertaken routinely in many centres. Echocardiography is essential if a complication of infarction is suspected such as ventricular septal rupture, papillary muscle dysfunction or left ventricular aneurysm. Stress echocardiography is an alternative to myocardial perfusion imaging for detecting ischaemia and viable myocardium in apparently infarcted regions.

Most commonly echocardiography is used preoperatively to assess ventricular function which is expressed as ejection fraction or fractional shortening. Valve abnormalities can be also be quantified. Whilst the majority of preoperative echoes are performed via the transthoracic route, approximately 15% of patients have poor acoustic windows and transoesophageal echocardiography (TOE) is required. This can be performed under sedation but many patients require general anaesthesia. The anaesthetist can gain valuable information from the echocardiogram report and, increasingly, cardiothoracic anaesthetists use TOE intraoperatively.

Cardiac catheterization and angiography

Cardiac catheterization is still considered the gold standard for diagnosis of cardiac pathology before surgery and is essential for the definition of lesions of the coronary vessels. Certain abnormalities, such as atrial or ventricular septal defect, and isolated valve lesions, can be adequately assessed using non-invasive means. However, a coronary angiogram is commonly undertaken in patients with apparently isolated valve lesions to ascertain if CABG is required. If only coronary anatomy is to be visualized, then a left heart study will be undertaken. If there is any degree of left ventricular dysfunction, valvular, abnormality or pulmonary disease, or right ventricular dysfunction, then a right heart study may also be performed.

Radio-opaque dye is injected through a catheter inserted via the femoral route and placed in the coronary ostia. The degree of vessel stenosis is assessed visually by the percentage reduction in diameter of the vessel, which correlates with the reduction in cross-sectional area at the point of narrowing. Lesions reducing vessel diameter by more than 50%, corresponding to a reduction in cross-sectional area of 75%, are considered significant.

Accurate intracardiac pressures can also be obtained. Left ventricular end-diastolic pressure is routinely measured and elevated values (> 15 mmHg) suggest ventricular impairment. An angiogram can be used to estimate ventricular function and ejection fraction. The latter is calculated from the difference in ventricular size between systole and diastole either manually or by computer. A normal ejection fraction is approximately 70% and, as this value drops with ventricular impairment, operative risk increases.

If valve lesions are present, it is usual to measure the gradient across the valve for stenotic lesions or to estimate the regurgitant fraction for valve incompetence. A relative scale of +1 to +4 is used to quantify the severity of valve incompetence during injection of the dye.

It is also possible to measure the oxygen saturation and oxygen content of the blood. If oxygen consumption is also measured, other variables, such as cardiac output, pulmonary to systemic flow ratios and pulmonary and systemic vascular resistance, can be calculated, these may be particularly important in the assessment of congenital lesions.

Interventional catheterization

Patients may have undergone angioplasty, or intracoronary stent insertion, some time before surgery. Occasionally, a patient may present as an emergency following a failed intervention, or with a complication, such

Table 1.8 Lesions which may in selected cases be treated in the catheter laboratory

Congenital pulmonary valve stenosis
Congenital aortic valve stenosis
Adult mitral valve stenosis
Closure of patent ductus arteriosus
Closure of atrial septal defect
Closure of ventricular septal defect
Hypertrophic obstructive cardiomyopathy
Certain types of arrhythmia (e.g. SVT, VT)

as a dissected coronary artery. Angioplasty entails balloon dilatation of a stenosed coronary artery and a stent may subsequently be inserted to maintain patency. Restenosis is common and multiple procedures may be undertaken before surgery is necessary. A number of other lesions can also be treated in the catheter laboratory (Table 1.8).

Computed tomography and cardiac magnetic resonance imaging

Computed tomography (CT) scanning may be used in the diagnosis of aortic dissections and other lesions of the thoracic aorta. It can be helpful before repeat surgery to ascertain the proximity of the heart to the sternum. Cardiac magnetic resonance imaging is being used increasingly and, unlike CT, it can be gated to the cardiac cycle allowing assessment of ventricular function. Magnetic resonance allows characterization of ischaemia and its extent.

Drug therapy
Anticoagulants
Aspirin
It has been shown that the anti-platelet effect of aspirin reduces mortality and infarction rates in unstable angina and significantly decreases mortality after acute myocardial infarction. Aspirin permanently inactivates the enzyme cyclo-oxygenase (COX) by acetylation, preventing formation of thromboxane A_2 and hence platelet aggregation. The duration of this effect is approximately the same as the lifetime of affected platelets in the circulation, 7–9 days. It is widely believed that aspirin therapy is associated with increased bleeding after cardiac surgery. As a result, in patients with stable coronary artery disease, it is usual to stop aspirin therapy at least 1 week before surgery to allow time for normally

functioning platelets to appear in the circulation. If the patient has unstable angina, or left mainstem stenosis, then it is safer to continue aspirin therapy until the day of surgery. Techniques to minimize bleeding include careful haemostasis, use of platelet concentrates and agents such as aprotinin which preserves platelet function. Aspirin improves graft patency after CABG and is often prescribed postoperatively.

Non-steroidal anti-inflammatory agents
Drugs such as diclofenac and ibuprofen also inhibit COX but the effect is reversible within 6–12 h. These drugs should also be stopped preoperatively, but the relationship between their use and postoperative bleeding is not well established.

Non-steroidal anti-inflammatory drugs (NSAIDs) have a number of other important side-effects, including gastrointestinal erosion and haemorrhage and renal impairment. The latter problem may be an interstitial nephritis associated with chronic ingestion of the drug or an acute effect resulting from prostaglandin inhibition in the kidney. Prostaglandin inhibition only has a marginal effect on renal perfusion in the normal kidney but, in circumstances of reduced renal perfusion, this influence may be profound. NSAIDs should be prescribed with caution in the elderly after surgery. If renal function is affected, then the drug should be withdrawn and empirical measures to preserve renal function instituted. The newer COX-2 inhibitors are considered to be less likely to cause bleeding and gastric irritation.

Warfarin
Warfarin is a synthetic coumarin derivative which acts by preventing formation of coagulation factors II, VII, IX and X in the liver by inhibition of vitamin K mediated gamma-carboxylation of precursor proteins. Patients presenting for surgery may be taking warfarin for a number of indications;

- Prosthetic valve *in situ*.
- Chronic atrial fibrillation.
- Previous pulmonary embolism.
- Risk of intracardiac thrombus.

The effect of warfarin is monitored by the prothrombin time but the recommended international normalized ratio (INR) varies. The onset of action of warfarin is delayed because clotting factors already synthesized must be cleared from the body and the peak effect does not occur for 36–72 h. Similarly, the half life is approximately 44 h and so warfarin is routinely withdrawn several days before surgery to reduce the INR to between 2 and 2.5. If there is particular concern, for example, in patients with prosthetic valves, then intravenous heparin is started to cover the operative period. If the INR remains high despite withdrawal of warfarin, then surgery may have to be postponed or the effect reversed by administration of vitamin K or infusion of fresh frozen plasma (FFP) (20 ml/kg). Vitamin K, takes up to 12 h to be effective and this may not be reflected in the coagulation profile for up to 24 h. More importantly, the effect is not reversible for up to 2 weeks. Thus, administration of FFP is preferable because it provides active coagulation factors with immediate effect. Furthermore, FFP may be required following cardiopulmonary bypass as transfused factors, especially factor VII, are cleared from the circulation more rapidly than the residual oral anticoagulant.

Heparin
Heparin is a complex organic acid derived from the lung, or liver, of domestic animals. Heparin compounds bind to the lycine-binding site of antithrombin III and increase its affinity for factor X several hundred fold. It also prevents fibrin clot formation by inhibiting thrombin-activated formation of fibrin stabilizing factor. The low molecular weight heparin molecules are responsible for the anticoagulant effect of most preparations. Heparin is used in the treatment of unstable angina, by infusion or regular subcutaneous injection, together with glyceryl trinitrate. Therapy should be continued until the loading dose of heparin is given before cardiopulmonary bypass. Paradoxically, heparin requirements may be increased in patients who are already receiving the drug, probably because of low levels of antithrombin III. This problem is usually overcome by increasing the bolus dose of heparin but, occasionally, administration of FFP is required to increase levels of circulating antithrombin III. Patients who have already received heparin can develop thrombocytopaenia as a result of antibodies to platelet receptors, so called heparin induced thrombocytopenia, which needs careful management. The platelet count falls as platelets are consumed during the formation of clots and emboli which can be fatal. An alternative anticoagulant, such as hirudin, will be required for cardiopulmonary bypass.

Thrombolytic agents
Thrombolytic agents, such as streptokinase and alteplase (tissue-type plasminogen activator), increase the amount of plasmin available to

break down fresh clot. They are used in the treatment of acute myocardial infarction (AMI) and have been associated with a reduction in
infarct size and improved outcome. They may reduce the incidence of
AMI in patients with unstable angina. Patients may present for surgery
after recent thrombolytic therapy usually associated with failed angioplasty or coronary stent insertion. Most of these drugs have a short half-
life (5–15 min) but may contribute to pathological bleeding in the
perioperative period. Use of clotting factors, such as FFP, platelets and
cryoprecipitate, may be necessary. Aminocaproic acid may be appropriate in these circumstances. Aprotinin, which inhibits fibrinolysis and
decreases production of fibrin degradation products during cardiopulmonary bypass, may also be indicated.

Newer anti-platelet agents
The pathogenesis of acute coronary ischaemia, occlusive stroke and
peripheral arterial occlusion usually involves platelet activation and
thrombosis. The final common pathway in platelet aggregation is the
binding of fibrinogen to activated GpIIb/IIIa receptors on adjacent
platelets. Specific murine antibodies to this membrane receptor have
been developed which prevent binding of fibrinogen and other ligands.
Some of these are now in therapeutic use and have been shown to be
beneficial as an adjunctive treatment for unstable angina and coronary
angioplasty. Abciximab (Reopro), tirofiban and eptifibatide are now
licensed for human use. In early trials, GpIIb/IIIa blockade was associated with significant bleeding complications but this was attributed to
concurrent therapy with heparin. Emergency bypass surgery following
the use of these agents was not complicated by excess bleeding.

Ticlopidine and clopidogrel prevent ADP-induced platelet aggregation. Both require hepatic transformation to an active metabolite. The
action appears to be permanent with antiplatelet activity lasting for
7–10 days. These drugs should be withdrawn 10–14 days before surgery
to minimize the risk of perioperative bleeding. In addition to effects on
platelet function and aggregation, these agents cause thrombocytopenia
and neutropenia, which occur in up to 2% of patients on long-term
therapy. Surgery should be postponed, if possible, if the white cell count
is low.

Cardiovascular drugs
With few exceptions, these drugs should be continued up to the day of
surgery. The main features of each drug group are presented in tabular
form, but the reader should consult standard texts for specific details.

Beta adrenoreceptor blocking agents
Beta blockade should be continued until the time of surgery to reduce perioperative ischaemia and hypertension and may be continued post-operatively. Excessive bradycardia can be treated with epicardial pacing. Atropine is rarely effective and isoprenaline reduces diastolic blood pressure and compromises coronary perfusion. Labetalol and metoprolol can be administered in the post-bypass period to control hypertension. Profound myocardial depression can occur in combination with calcium antagonists. The advantages and disadvantages of beta blockers are shown in Table 1.9.

Nitrates
Nitroglycerin is a smooth muscle relaxant and the mechanism of action is via nitric oxide. Therapy should be continued up to the time of surgery. Although widely used by cardiac anaesthetists, the value of prophylactic nitroglycerin in reducing intraoperative ischaemia remains controversial. The advantages and disadvantages of these drugs are shown in Table 1.10.

Calcium channel blockers
Nifedipine is a potent arterial dilator used to treat hypertension, whilst verapamil slows atrioventricular nodal conduction and is used to treat arrhythmias. Diltiazem is less negatively inotropic and the reduced

---

Table 1.9   Advantages and disadvantages of beta blocker therapy

Advantages	Disadvantages
Used to treat angina, hypertension, arrhythmias	May cause excessive bradycardia
Reduced mortality after acute myocardial infarction	Myocardial depression
Specific actions of different drugs variable	Can mask signs of hypoglycaemia
Reduced heart rate and contractility	Abrupt withdrawal dangerous
Reduced outflow obstruction in hypertrophic obstructive cardiomyopathy	Interactions with other drugs
May improve symptoms in left ventricular failure	C/I asthma, peripheral vascular disease
Prophylaxis for postoperative arrhythmias	Excretion impaired by renal/ liver disease

Table 1.10   Advantages and disadvantages of nitrates

Advantages	Disadvantages
Used to treat angina and heart failure	May produce hypotension
Coronary vasodilation	May cause methaemoglobinaemia
Improved collateral blood flow	
Reduced cardiac filling pressures	
Reduced myocardial oxygen demand	
Variable routes of administration	
Pulmonary vasodilator	

systemic vascular resistance is associated with improved cardiac output. These agents should not be withdrawn preoperatively unless there are signs of myocardial failure or a long PR interval on the ECG. The advantages and disadvantages of calcium channel blockade are shown in Table 1.11

Angiotensin-converting enzyme inhibitors
It has been suggested that the use of angiotensin-converting enzyme (ACE) inhibitors is associated with profound hypotension during cardiopulmonary bypass. The evidence is conflicting but these drugs are commonly withdrawn 24–48 h before surgery. The advantages and disadvantages of ACE inhibitors are shown in Table 1.12.

Table 1.11   Advantages and disadvantages of calcium channel blockade

Advantages	Disadvantages
Used to treat angina, hypertension and arrhythmias	Negatively inotropic
Heterogeneous effects on cardiovascular system	Slow atrioventricular nodal conduction
Reduced myocardial oxygen demand	May cause profound hypotension
Coronary vasodilation	Interaction with other drugs
Arterial dilation	No intravenous formulation in UK
Prevent spasm in arterial conduits	

Table 1.12   Advantages and disadvantages of angiotensin-converting enzyme inhibition

Advantages	Disadvantages
Reduced mortality from heart failure, cerebrovascular accident, myocardial infarction	May cause hyperkalaemia
Used to treat hypertension	Hypotension
Increased stroke volume, cardiac output	May impair renal function
	Hypotension during cardiopulmonary bypass
	Cough

Other drugs that have important cardiovascular effects include Losartan, which is a non-peptide antagonist of the angiotensin receptor. It exerts an antihypertensive effect, lasting 24 h, and is highly effective in combination with low dose diuretics. Nicorandil is a potassium channel activator, combined with a nitrate, used in the treatment of angina. It relaxes smooth muscle causing dilatation of both diseased and normal coronary arteries. It has no effect on myocardial contractility or heart rate, and is beneficial in reducing both pre- and after-load. It can be used safely with other anti-anginals, digoxin and frusemide. Nicorandil is potentially cardioprotective in the perioperative period and may reduce postischaemia reperfusion injury.

Anti-dysrhythmic drugs, diuretics and lipid lowering agents
Drugs in these groups are not generally withdrawn before surgery and may be continued postoperatively. Lipid lowering agents are often not restarted until the patients is discharged or seen in outpatients. Binding of digoxin may be affected by cardiopulmonary bypass and, previously, it was withdrawn a few days preoperatively. If digoxin levels are within the therapeutic range, then this is not necessary. Amiodarone is commonly used in the treatment of atrial and ventricular arrhythmias. It should be used with caution in patients on beta blockers. It increases the free plasma digoxin concentration and potentiates the action of warfarin. Patients on long-term amiodarone therapy may have abnormal thyroid function, which should be checked preoperatively.

Many patients will be taking diuretics, which may result in abnormal serum electrolyte values. Excessive diuresis causes hypovolaemia with elevated urea and creatinine levels. Hypovolaemia makes the patient sensitive to vasodilation produced by anaesthetic agents, with the risk of profound hypotension on induction. Patients on diuretics preoperatively usually require them in the early postoperative period.

Hypoglycaemic agents
Diabetic patients presenting for cardiac surgery can be managed using principles applicable to other forms of major surgery carried out under general anaesthesia.

The sulphonylurea group of hypoglycaemic agents act as potassium channel blockers, which may counteract any beneficial effects of ischaemic preconditioning. This may contribute to the increased mortality and morbidity seen in diabetic patients after cardiac surgery.

Premedication
Traditionally 'heavy' premedication was prescribed to prevent ischaemia during induction of anaesthesia and reduce anxiety induced sympathetic stimulation of the cardiovascular system. Improved cardiovascular control with modern drugs has made this approach unnecessary. Concerns about respiratory depression with opiates and the need for early extubation has led anaesthetists to use fewer sedative agents for premedication. Benzodiazepines, such as temazepam, are commonly used. This drug can be given orally 1–2 h before surgery with the dose being repeated if surgery is delayed. Particularly anxious patients may be given a dose of longer acting agents, such as diazepam or lorazepam, the night before surgery.

Antibiotic prophylaxis
Prophylactic antibiotics are given to all patients undergoing cardiac surgery. The first dose should be given in the anaesthetic room, ideally before bladder catheterization, particularly in patients with valve abnormalities. Dosage regimens and the choice of agents vary between units. Theoretically, effective surgical prophylaxis only requires adequate tissue levels of the drug at the time of the operation.

Further reading
Chapeau I. Grading of angina pectoris. Circulation 1975;54:522.
Dupuis J-Y, Wang F, Nathan H, Lam M, Grimes S, Bourke M. The Cardiac Anesthesia Risk Evaluation Score. Anesthesiology 2001;94:194–204.
EPIC Investigators. Use of monoclonal antibody directed against platelet Glycoprotein IIb/IIIa receptor in high-risk coronary angioplasty. N Engl J Med 1994;330:956–961.

EPILOG Investigators. Platelet IIb/IIIa receptor blockade and low dose heparin during percutaneous coronary revascularisation. N Engl J Med 1997;336: 1689–1696.

Nashef SA, Roques F, Michel P, Gauducheau E, Lemeshow S, Salamon R. European system for cardiac operative risk evaluation (EuroSCORE). Eur J Cardiothorac Surg 1999;16:9–13.

National Adult Cardiac Surgical Database Report 1999–2000. London: The Society of Cardiothoracic Surgeons of Great Britain and Ireland; 2000.

Parsonnet V, Dean D, Bernstein AD. A method of uniform stratification of risk for evaluating the results of surgery in acquired adult heart disease. Circulation 1989;79(suppl 1):1.3–1.12.

Pigott D, Nagle C, Allman K, Westaby S, Evans R. Effect of omitting regular ACE inhibitor medication before cardiac surgery on haemodynamic variables and vasoactive drug requirements. Br J Anaesth 1999;83:715–720.

Topol E, Byzova T, Plow E. Platelet GPIIb/IIIa blockers. Lancet 1999; 353:227–231.

Turner J, Morgan C, Thakrar B, Pepper J. Difficulties in predicting outcome in cardiac surgery. Crit Care Med 1995;23:1843–1850.

Vuylsteke A, Oduro A, Cardan E, Latimer R. Effect of aspirin in coronary artery bypass grafting. J Cardiothorac Vasc Anaesth 1997;11:832–834.

2

Anaesthesia for cardiac surgery

There are now a number of techniques that can be used effectively to provide anaesthesia for patients undergoing cardiac surgery. However, there is substantial evidence that it is not the choice of anaesthetic technique, or group of drugs, that is selected, but the manner in which they are used which is important. The requirement to maintain myocardial oxygen balance remains, but a number of other factors must be considered, including the desire for early extubation, concerns about silent myocardial ischaemia and new approaches to pain management. Provided the anaesthetist is cognizant of the principles involved and intervenes to interrupt adverse haemodynamic changes, then any anaesthetic agents can be used safely. The anaesthetic technique may influence the end result but the patient's primary disease, operative technique and inadequate myocardial preservation are more important determinants of outcome.

A detailed description of all available agents and their pharmacology is beyond the scope of this book. A description of the different techniques used and some of the possible advantages and disadvantages are discussed. The relevant cardiovascular effects of the major induction agents, volatile agents and neuromuscular blocking agents are tabulated. This chapter provides a general approach to monitoring, induction, maintenance and haemodynamic management for adult cardiac surgery. Specific operations and clinical situations are described in more detail in Chapter 4.

Monitoring

The Association of Cardiothoracic Anaesthetists have recently published guidelines about standards of monitoring of both the patient and the extracorporeal circuit. Standard monitoring for cardiac surgery is shown in Table 2.1. Non-invasive monitoring should be attached to the patient before induction. In addition, invasive arterial monitoring is advisable and, in some units, central venous lines are also inserted under local anaesthetic before induction of anaesthesia.

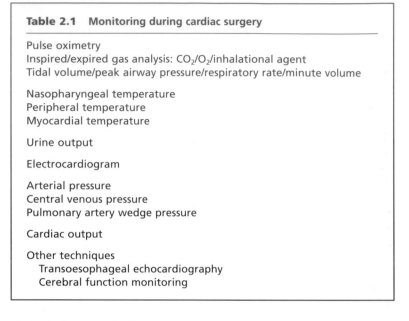

Table 2.1   Monitoring during cardiac surgery

Pulse oximetry
Inspired/expired gas analysis: CO_2/O_2/inhalational agent
Tidal volume/peak airway pressure/respiratory rate/minute volume

Nasopharyngeal temperature
Peripheral temperature
Myocardial temperature

Urine output

Electrocardiogram

Arterial pressure
Central venous pressure
Pulmonary artery wedge pressure

Cardiac output

Other techniques
    Transoesophageal echocardiography
    Cerebral function monitoring

Arterial cannulation

Anaesthesia for cardiac surgery is frequently associated with rapid and sudden changes in blood pressure and a safe and reliable method of measuring acute changes continuously is required. Preinduction insertion of a radial artery cannula in the non-dominant hand (usually the left) is advisable, and is mandatory in high-risk cases such as aortic stenosis, left mainstem coronary disease and patients with poor ventricular function. The advantages and disadvantages of radial artery cannulation are shown in Table 2.2.

Table 2.2   Advantages and disadvantages of using the radial artery for invasive monitoring during cardiac surgery

Advantages	Disadvantages
Easy to cannulate	Radial artery may be needed as a conduit
Accessible during surgery	Sternal retractor may compress radial artery
Good collateral circulation	
Low incidence of complications	
Easy to inspect for ischaemia	

The right radial artery may be preferred if aortic surgery is to be undertaken, or if an intra-aortic balloon pump (IABP) is to be inserted. Other arteries can be used including brachial, axillary, femoral or dorsalis pedis arteries. The femoral artery may be required for insertion of an IABP or to institute cardiopulmonary bypass in repeat surgery and the trace from the dorsalis pedis artery may be compromised in low output states or if the patient is cold.

Central venous access

Peripheral venous access will have been established before induction and a large bore cannula can be sited in the arm for volume replacement during surgery. Central venous access is required:

- To measure central venous pressure.
- For the administration of vasoactive drugs.
- To float a pulmonary artery catheter.
- To pass a transvenous pacing wire, if required postoperatively.

The right internal jugular vein is commonly used for the following reasons:

- It can usually be palpated and is easy to cannulate.
- It can be imaged with ultrasound, if necessary.
- Low incidence of complications.
- Pressure recordings are not affected if the innominate vein is stretched on opening the chest.
- Multiple catheters can be placed in the same vessel.

A higher approach to the internal jugular vein is preferable, because pneumothorax and damage to vascular structures within the chest is less likely. The Seldinger technique is safe and widely practised, although complications relating to over zealous use of the dilator have been described. Puncture of the carotid artery with a small needle is not usually serious but, if this is undetected or a large sheath is passed into the vessel, then surgical repair may be necessary. The subclavian vein is an alternative, but it is more hazardous. For patients undergoing combined carotid endarterectomy and coronary artery bypass grafting (CABG), the subclavian approach may be preferable.

Cardiac output monitoring

Thermodilution remains the 'gold standard' for clinical determination of cardiac output, but use of pulmonary artery catheters (PACS) remains controversial. In a recent editoral, Leibowitz stated that: 'after reviewing the available evidence placing a pulmonary artery catheter in patients undergoing straightforward coronary artery bypass grafting has been shown in a single large study not to change outcome and use of pulmonary artery catheters in this setting appears to be dictated by regional and personal preference'. (From Liebowitz AB 1998)

In selected cases, such as patients with poor ventricular function or valve disease, PAC may facilitate the choice of inotropes. A PAC may also be useful in the management of patients with significant pulmonary hypertension. Our practice is to routinely insert a PAC sheath following induction of anaesthesia. A PAC can then be introduced quickly, if required, at the termination of cardiopulmonary bypass (CPB) or once the patient reaches the intensive care unit.

Pulmonary artery catheterization allows measurement of pulmonary artery pressure, pulmonary capillary wedge pressure and thermodilution cardiac output, and mixed venous oxygen saturation. More sophisticated devices are available which can measure cardiac

Table 2.3 Indices that may be derived from pulmonary artery catheter data

Cardiac output	CO
Cardiac index	CI = CO/body surface area (BSA)
Stroke volume	SV = CO/heart rate
Stroke volume index	SVI = SV/BSA
Pulmonary vascular resistance	PVR = [mean pulmonary artery pressure – mean pulmonary capillary wedge pressure (PCWP)] × 80/CO
Systemic vascular resistance	SVR = [mean blood pressure (BP) – mean right atrial pressure (RAP)] × 80/CO
Left ventricular stroke work	LVSW = SV × (mean BP – mean PCWP) × 0.0136
LVSW index	LVSWI = SVI × (mean BP – mean RAP) × 0.0136

Normal values
CI = 2.5–4.2 l/min/m^2
SVI = 30–65 ml/beat/m^2
PVR = 150–250 dynes/s/cm^5
SVR = 700–1600 dynes/s/cm^5

output continuously and some have a pacing facility. A variety of haemodynamic indices can be calculated from these data (Table 2.3) in conjunction with measurements of systolic and diastolic arterial pressure and central venous pressure. Much information can also be gained by observing the contraction and filling state of the right and left heart and the pulmonary artery without recourse to invasive monitoring. Data from PACs should be viewed with caution in patients with mitral valve disease or in whom positive end-expiratory pressure is being used.

Insertion of pulmonary artery catheters is associated with a number of complications (Table 2.4). Less invasive methods of monitoring cardiac output are shown in Table 2.5.

Table 2.4   Complications of pulmonary artery catheterization

Arrhythmias
Malposition
Pulmonary artery rupture
Right ventricular rupture
Tricuspid/pulmonary valve damage
Catheter knotting
Thrombosis/embolism
Pneumothorax/vascular damage during insertion
Infection

Transoesophageal echocardiography

The use of intraoperative echocardiography during cardiac surgery is becoming widespread. Increasingly, anaesthetists are undergoing training in echocardiography and use the device as an intraoperative monitor. Transoesophageal echocardiography is now regarded as an essential monitor during valve surgery and repair of congenital defects. It is also useful to facilitate weaning from cardiopulmonary bypass (CPB) when difficulties arise and for detection of regional wall motion abnormalities following coronary artery surgery.

Neurological monitoring

Significant neurological injury in the form of stroke occurs in approximately 1% to 3% of patients, but more subtle neuropsychological deficits are detectable in up to 70% of patients. Risk factors for neurological injury include:

Table 2.5 Continuous cardiac output monitors

Monitor	Technique	Comments
Oesophageal Doppler	Doppler ultrasound	Simple Minimally invasive Useful trend analysis Real time haemodynamic display Visual representation of aortic blood flow, preload, afterload and contracility User dependent Frequent repositioning Variable correlation with thermodilution Diathermy interference Patient must be anaesthetized Need estimate of aortic diameter No pressure measurementts
$NICO_2$	Differential CO_2 Fick partial rebreathing	Good correlation with thermodilution Limited clinical experience Minimally invasive
LiDCO	Pulse contour analysis Lithium dilution	Uses existing arterial and venous access Use on awake patients Validated against thermodilution No diathermy/electrical interference Recalibration required after 8–12 h Real time haemodynamic display No intracardiac pressure measurements
Thoracic bioimpedance	Measurement of thoracic electrical impedance	Unreliable in critically ill patients Hostile electrical environment in theatre Limited use in cardiac disease Correct lead placement essential Non-invasive Affected by pulmonary oedema Inaccurate with intracardiac shunts Need to estimate thoracic length No pressure measurements

- Advanced age.
- Proximal aortic atheroma.
- Diabetes mellitus.
- Previous stroke or transient ischaemic attack.
- Pulmonary disease.
- Previous cardiac surgery.
- Unstable angina.

Considerable effort has been directed towards reducing the incidence of neurological complications. Despite technological advances in neurological monitoring, each technique has a number of inherent difficulties which reduces its usefulness.

Electroencephalography (EEG) is considered the gold standard for detection of cerebral ischaemia. Monitoring via scalp electrodes is cumbersome, requires expert interpretation and electrical interference is common. There is a weak association between EEG deficits and early neuropsychometric outcome after CPB.

Transcranial Doppler is a non-invasive technique using Doppler ultrasound to measure cerebral blood flow velocity in the middle cerebral artery. It can detect emboli and newer devices can discriminate between gaseous and particulate matter. The number of emboli detected intraoperatively has been correlated with neurological deficits appearing postoperatively.

Jugular venous bulb oxygen saturation (SjVO$_2$) monitoring is an invasive technique used to measure cerebral venous oxygen saturation. A catheter is passed percutaneously into the jugular vein and positioned with its tip in the jugular bulb. Measurements are made intermittently with a co-oximeter or continuously via a fibreoptic catheter. A reduction in SjVO$_2$ represents an imbalance between oxygen supply (cerebral blood flow) and demand (cerebral metabolic rate). The relationship between SjVO$_2$ desaturation and postoperative neuropsychological deficit is controversial.

Near-infrared spectroscopy has been used to monitor cerebral oxygenation and indirectly measures cerebral blood flow. The principle is similar to pulse oximetry. It has been widely used in neonates but its role in CPB is less well defined.

Induction of anaesthesia

After appropriate monitoring has been established and preoxygenation completed, induction of anaesthesia is commenced via the intravenous route. A common approach is to administer a moderate dose of opioid (fentanyl 5–10 μg/kg, alfentanil 50–100 μg/kg or remifentanil 1 μg/kg) before a sleep dose of etomidate, thiopentone or propofol given by slow injection. This provides a smooth induction with haemodynamic stability. Pretreatment with opioids reduces the dose of induction agent required and decreases the myocardial depression and fall in systemic vascular resistance associated with them.

The cardiovascular effects of commonly used induction agents are shown in Table 2.6. Etomidate is widely used for induction because it has minimal cardiovascular effects in normal subjects, but reductions in blood pressure do occur in patients with cardiac disease or some degree of hypovolaemia.

Alternative approaches include the use of benzodiazepines. Cardiovascular stability is well maintained with diazemuls and it may be used to facilitate insertion of invasive monitoring lines under local anaesthetic. Midazolam may cause hypotension at induction due to falls in systemic vascular resistance and stroke volume, particularly in combination with opioids. Ketamine produces a substantial rise in arterial pressure as a result of sympathetic stimulation. This may be advantageous; for example, in the patient with a large pericardial effusion presenting for drainage.

Muscular relaxation

After induction of anaesthesia, the trachea is intubated following the administration of a non-depolarizing muscle relaxant. The cardiovascular effects of commonly used muscle relaxants are shown in Table 2.7.

Pancuronium is widely used by cardiac anaesthetists because its sympathomimetic and vagolytic actions are considered advantageous. However, these effects produce an increase in myocardial oxygen demand which could result in ischaemia, particularly in association with

Table 2.6   Cardiovascular effects of commonly used induction agents

Drug	Heart rate	Stroke–volume ratio	Cardiac output	Mean arterial pressure
Thiopentone	Increase	Increase	Decrease	Decrease
Etomidate	Increase	Decrease	Unchanged	Unchanged
Propofol	Unchanged	Decrease	Decrease	Decrease

Table 2.7 Cardiovascular effects of commonly used muscle relaxants

Drug	Heart rate	Stroke–volume ratio	Cardiac output	Mean arterial pressure
Pancuronium	Increase	Increase	Increase	Increase
Vecuronium	Unchanged	Unchanged	Unchanged	Unchanged
Rocuronium	Increase	Unchanged	Unchanged	Unchanged
Atracurium	Unchanged	Unchanged	Unchanged	Unchanged

the stress response to intubation. Use of beta adrenergic receptor blockers limits the severity of the tachycardia and hypertension.

Vecuronium with a shorter half life, and stable cardiovascular profile is used increasingly, but may be associated with bradycardia if given shortly after fentanyl or remifentanil. Rocuronium has a similar haemo-dynamic profile and its rapid onset facilitates early intubation.

Atracurium, as a continuous infusion, may be useful for short non-bypass procedures, but histamine release can cause hypotension.

Tracheal intubation

The tracheal is usually intubated via the oral route. Nasal intubation may cause mucosal trauma resulting in severe haemorrhage following administration of heparin. Certain procedures require use of double lumen endobronchial tubes (Table 2.8).

Use of a double lumen tube allows collapse of the lung on the oper-ative side to facilitate surgery. A left-sided tube is usually selected to circumvent problems associated with right upper lobe ventilation. Placement of the tube must be undertaken with great care and prefer-ably using a fibreoptic scope to ensure correct positioning.

Table 2.8 Operations that may require use of a double lumen tube

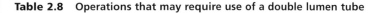

Repair of descending thoracic aortic aneurysm
Repeat mitral valve surgery
Repair of adult coarctation of the aorta
Beating heart coronary artery surgery via left thoracotomy
Adult modified Blalock–Taussig shunt

Maintenance of anaesthesia

The aim of anaesthesia for cardiac surgery is to maintain myocardial oxygen balance and minimize ischaemia. Ischaemia may be avoided if hypertension leading to increased wall-tension and tachycardia are avoided. Anaesthetic or analgesics agents alone rarely provide complete haemodynamic control and additional drug therapy with a variety of vasoactive agents, including nitrates, vasoconstrictors and inotropes, may be required. A typical anaesthetic technique is the combination of an opioid and a volatile agent. Total intravenous anaesthesia is also widely used such as a propofol/opioid combination.

The use of nitrous oxide in cardiac anaesthesia is controversial. It has myocardial depressant effects which may be enhanced if used in combination with opiates. An air/oxygen mix should be used as the carrier gas for volatile agents. The cardiovascular effects of volatile agents are shown in Table 2.9.

A range of synthetic opioids are available. Fentanyl and two of its newer congeners, alfentanil and sufentanil, are effective in cardiac anaesthesia with minimal cardiovascular depression. Remifentanil, a potent agent with, an ultra short half life (5 min) resulting from metabolism by plasma esterases, is administered by infusion at a rate of 1–2 μg/kg/min. Remifentanil has been successfully used with both propofol and isoflurane to provide intraoperative haemodynamic stability during cardiac surgery. Patients can usually be extubated within 30 min of discontinuing the infusion.

Neuraxial blockade

Two techniques have been used to provide intraoperative analgesia during cardiac surgery, intrathecal opiates and continuous epidural infusion of a low-dose local anaesthetic/opioid combination. Intrathecal

---

Table 2.9   Cardiovascular effects of volatile anaesthetic agents

Drug	Heart rate	Stroke–volume ratio	Cardiac output	Mean arterial pressure
Isoflurane	Increase	Decrease	Maintained	Decrease
Enflurane	Increase	Decrease	Decrease	Decrease
Sevoflurane	Unchanged	Unchanged	Maintained	Unchanged
Desflurane	Increase	Increase	Maintained	Increase
Halothane	Unchanged	Decrease	Decrease	Decrease

morphine provides good intraoperative and early postoperative analgesia but often results in respiratory depression, which delays extubation.

In addition to excellent analgesia, thoracic epidural analgesia (TEA) may improve the outcome of patients undergoing CABG surgery through cardiac sympatholysis and CPB-related stress response attenuation.

TEA improves myocardial oxygen balance in number of ways:

● Selective vasodilation of atherosclerotic segments.
● Decreased coronary vascular resistance for collateral flow.
● Redistribution of blood to the subendocardium.
● Maintained cardiac output, stroke–volume ratio and coronary perfusion pressure.

TEA is associated with a reduction in the incidence of hypertension during bypass with fewer pharmacological interventions required. TEA provides excellent analgesia, with improved respiratory function and smoother control of blood pressure in the postoperative period. This technique may be associated with hypotension and bradycardia

TEA has the potential to cause an epidural haematoma with paralysis. The optimal time for epidural catheter insertion is unknown but, for safety, several hours should elapse between insertion and heparin administration. The place of TEA in cardiac anaesthesia is hotly debated.

Further reading

Arrowsmith J, Grocott H, Newman M. Neurologic risk assessment, monitoring and outcome in cardiac surgery. J Cardiothorac Vasc Anaesth 1999;13: 736–743.

Liebowitz AB. Perioperative Pulmonary Artery Catheterisation: what is the evidence that it improves outcome? J Cardiothoracic Vasc Anaesth 1998 Feb; 12(1):3–9.

Liem TH, Booij LH, Hasenbos MA, Gielen MJM. Coronary artery bypass using two different anaesthetic techniques. J Cardiothorac Vasc Anaesth 1992; 6:148–116.

Meissner A, Rolf N, Van Aken H. Thoracic epidural anesthesia and the patient with heart disease: benefits, risks and controversies. Anesth Analg 1997;85:517–528.

Mora C, Dudek C, Torjman M, White PF. The effects of anesthetic technique on the hemodynamic response and recovery profile in coronary revascularization patients. Anesth Analg 1995;81:900–910.

Sanchez R, Nygard E. Epidural anaesthesia in cardiac surgery: is there an increased risk? J Cardiothorac Vasc Anesth 1998;12:170–173.

Slogoff S, Keats A. Randomised trial of primary anaesthetic agents on outcome of coronary artery bypass operations. Anesthesiology 1989;70:179–188.

Stump D, Jones TJJ, Rorie Kashemi. Neurophysiologic monitoring and outcomes in cardiovascular surgery. J Cardiothorac Vasc Anesth 1999; 13:600–613.

3

Anaesthesia for 'beating heart' coronary artery bypass grafting

Coronary artery surgery on a beating heart was first described in the 1960s. However, the development of cardiopulmonary bypass (CPB) and cardioplegic techniques facilitated rapid advances in coronary artery surgery by providing a motionless, bloodless surgical field. Renewed interest in beating heart coronary artery surgery (BHCAS) resulted from recognition of the deleterious effects of extracorporeal circuits, a desire for less invasive surgery and the need to reduce health-care costs and re-evaluate hospital resources. The potential advantages of BHCAS are shown in Table 3.1.

Optimizing conditions for surgery, whilst maintaining haemo-dynamic stability during cardiac displacement, is essential. Enhancing myocardial protection by early detection and treatment of ischaemia may reduce myocardial injury and improve outcome. Whilst basic care of the patient is similar to that for conventional coronary artery bypass grafting (CABG), there are some important differences.

Surgical approach
In an attempt to reduce invasiveness, a number of incisions other than sternotomy have been used. Left anterior thoracotomy for left internal

---

Table 3.1 Potential advantages of beating heart coronary artery surgery

Reduced inflammatory response
Reduced neurological injury
Reduced renal impairment
Reduced incidence of coagulopathy
Reduced transfusion requirements
Avoidance of hypothermia
Shorter intensive care unit and hospital stay
Reduced cost

mammary (LIMA) to left anterior descending coronary artery (LAD) anastomosis was popular initially, the so-called minimally invasive direct coronary artery bypass (MIDCAB). Difficulties with access through limited incisions have led to median sternotomy being the option currently favoured by most surgeons for multivessel surgery and termed off-pump coronary artery bypass (OPCAB). Advances in robotic assisted surgery using thoracoscopic ports may mean that a number of small incisions is all that is required. The advantages and disadvantages of these approaches are shown in Table 3.2.

Patient selection

Initial attention focused on patients with single- or two-vessel disease, unsuitable for percutaneous transluminal coronary angioplasty or stent

Table 3.2   Advantages and disadvantages of different incisions for beating heart coronary artery surgery

Median sternotomy

Advantages:	Disadvantages:
Familiar	Large incision
Access to all vessels	Sternal and mediastinal infections
Well tolerated	Risks with repeat surgery
Avoids rib damage	
Easy conversion to cardiopulmonary bypass	

Left thoracotomy

Advantages:	Disadvantages:
Reduced morbidity	Limited access
	Painful incision
	Excessive retraction required
	Reports of partial breast necrosis from retractors
	Risk of rib damage
	Risk of chronic pain syndromes

Endoscopic approach

Advantages:	Disadvantages:
Minimally invasive	Limited access
Rapid recovery	View may be obscured by bleeding
	One-lung ventilation required
	Robotic systems unfamiliar
	Only suitable for left internal mammary to left anterior descending coronary artery graft

procedures, who had good ventricular function and low comorbidity. The scope of BHCAS has expanded to include patients with more extensive disease, poor ventricular function and those requiring repeat surgery, and also patients with cerebrovascular disease, renal failure and chronic lung disease who might benefit from avoiding CPB. Relative contraindications are shown in Table 3.3. One important goal of BHCAS is to reduce blood loss and hence transfusion requirements.

Preoperative assessment and premedication

Detailed preoperative assessment is essential and similar to that for patients undergoing conventional CABG surgery, as discussed in Chapter 1. A history of congestive heart failure, arrhythmias and unstable angina may be contraindications. If one-lung ventilation (OLV) is planned, then careful evaluation of respiratory function should be undertaken.

Baseline electrocardiogram (ECG) and echocardiographic data should be recorded. The anaesthetist should review the angiogram, and this may help to predict the degree of haemodynamic compromise that will occur during coronary artery occlusion. If the patient has poor ventricular function, then preoperative insertion of an intra-aortic balloon pump should be considered.

Table 3.3   Relative contraindications to beating heart coronary artery surgery

Atrial fibrillation
Loss of normal atrial contraction may contribute to low cardiac output and increased heart rate making surgery difficult

Ventricular arrhythmias
Reappearance during surgery may be associated with profound reduction of cardiac output.

Congestive cardiac failure
Large heart is difficult to manipulate and haemodynamic changes accentuated.

Valvular disease
May make the patient less tolerant of low heart rate and manipulation of the heart

Chronic lung disease
May not be able to tolerate one-lung ventilation for MIDCAB

Cardiac medication should be continued until the morning of surgery. It is not necessary to stop angiotensin-converting enzyme inhibitors early and it may be desirable to continue nicorandil because it has myocardial protective properties. Most patients are already taking beta blockers, and although current stabilization devices have made routine use unnecessary, a single dose of atenolol on the morning of surgery can be helpful.

Premedication varies with the planned anaesthetic technique. Although benzodiazepines are popular, clonidine can contribute to reducing heart rate intraoperatively and augment postoperative analgesia. If a thoracic epidural is part of the anaesthetic technique, this should be performed several hours before surgery to minimize the risk of haematoma formation.

Anaesthetic technique

The aims of anaesthesia for BHCAS are shown in Table 3.4. The opportunity to 'fast track' these patients by avoiding hypothermia makes extubation possible in the operating room or shortly after completion of surgery. The desire for early extubation must not detract from maintaining adequate depth of anaesthesia. Patients with extensive comorbidity may not be suitable for early extubation. Many centres use an opiate-based technique, fentanyl sufentanil and remifentanil have been used. Volatile agents are commonly used for maintenance and isoflurane may have a myocardial protective effect during ischaemia. Total intravenous anaesthesia with propofol and opiates is also suitable. Although pancuronium is often used for neuromuscular blockade in BHCAS, some prefer vecuronium because of its tendency to produce bradycardia and its shorter half-life.

Thoracic epidura analgesia (TEA) is a theoretically attractive option for BHCAS. TEA at T3/T4 produces cardiac sympatholysis with selective vasodilation of atheromatous coronary artery segments,

---

Table 3.4   Aims of anaesthesia for beating heart coronary artery surgery

To facilitate surgery
To maintain haemodynamic stability
To maximize myocardial protection
To provide good postoperative analgesia

decreased resistance to collateral flow and redistribution of blood to the subendocardium. TEA may alleviate coronary steal and provides excellent haemodynamic stability, reducing hypertension whilst maintaining cardiac output, systemic vascular resistance and coronary perfusion pressure. Use of TEA permits early extubation, provides good postoperative analgesia and possibly reduces postoperative ischaemia and the incidence of arrhythmias.

If OLV is required for MIDCAB, or thoracoscopic harvest of the internal mammary artery, then an appropriately sized double-lumen tube (DLT) must be inserted. As hypoxia resulting from malposition of the DLT is highly undesirable in patients with ischaemic heart disease, the position of the tube should be confirmed by fibreoptic bronchoscopy before surgery starts. Insufflation of carbon dioxide into the operative haemothorax may be used in addition to OLV. An insufflation pressure of 10 mmHg or greater can cause significant haemodynamic instability.

Monitoring

The appropriate level of monitoring for patients undergoing BHCAS is controversial. Initial concern about ischaemic ventricular function prompted the use of transoesophageal echocardiography (TOE) and a pulmonary artery catheter (PAC) in addition to standard invasive monitoring. However, much BHCAS is undertaken on patients with good ventricular function undergoing one- or two-vessel surgery in whom extensive monitoring is unnecessary. When multiple grafts are contemplated in patients with impaired left ventricular function, a PAC may be useful. TOE provides immediate and specific information about ventricular function during coronary occlusion and after graft completion. The limitations of monitoring modalities during BHCAS are shown in Table 3.5.

A number of 'less invasive' continuous cardiac output monitoring devices are now available. These include oesophageal Doppler, partial carbon dioxide rebreathing, thoracic bioimpedance and pulse contour analysis.

In conclusion, if preoperative discussion with the surgeon indicates a brief procedure in a patient with good ventricular function, then five-lead ECG with ST segment analysis, an arterial line and a central venous catheter is probably adequate monitoring. At the other extreme, multivessel grafting in a high risk patient with poor left ventricular function might warrant use of TOE and a pulmonary artery catheter.

Table 3.5 Monitoring for beating heart coronary artery surgery

Monitor	Advantages	Disadvantages
Electrocardiogram	Simple Routine II and V5 good ischaemia detection ST segment analysis possible	Vectors change with position of heart Insensitive for ischaemia
Central venous pressure	Simple Routine	No help with ischaemia detection Affected by patient position
Pulmonary artery catheter	Can measure pulmonary artery wedge pressure, cardiac output Can measure mixed venous oxygen May have pacing facility	Insensitive for ischaemia Repositioning required if heart moved May generate arrhythmias Frequent complications May not be continuous
Transoesophageal echocardiography	Very sensitive for ischaemia Good indicator of function Indicates filling status	Expensive Trained user required View obscured when heart lifted

Stabilization techniques

The main challenge of BHCAS has been to produce complete revascularization with minimal myocardial damage, good long-term results and reproducibility, whilst operating on a moving target. A number of techniques have been developed to stabilize the operative field. A pharmacological approach was used initially with a range of drugs including beta blockers, adenosine and calcium antagonists (Table 3.6.). The use of drugs to slow the heart is controversial because these agents often depress ventricular function. Paradoxically, when the heart rate is slow, there may be more movement in the surgical field because of the increase in stroke volume.

A variety of mechanical stabilizers are now available and these have reduced the need for heart rate control. The most widely used is the Octopus device (Medtronic, Watford, UK). This instrument consists of two parallel paddles each with 4/5 suction domes. The paddles are placed parallel to the artery to be grafted to maintain maximum immobilization with minimum compromise of myocardial function. Once fixed in position with negative suction applied (approximately –500 mmHg) to the domes, the motion of the target artery is minimal.

Haemodynamic control

Some degree of haemodynamic disturbance occurs during the various manoeuvres required to bring the target vessel into view, and during

Table 3.6 Drugs used to produce bradycardia during beating heart coronary artery surgery

Drug	Advantages	Disadvantages
Esmolol (beta blocker)	Cardioselective Half-life 9 min Bolus/infusion suitable	Negative inotrope Tachyphylaxis Pacing required to reverse effect
Adenosine (endogenous nucleoside)	Half life 10 s Multiple boluses well tolerated Potentiated by dypiridamole	Produces asystole May cause hypotension May cause bronchospasm
Diltiazem (calcium antagonist)	Coronary vasodilatation Increases collateral flow No effect on contractility Useful for arterial conduits	No intravenous formulation in UK

periods of ischaemia induced by temporary coronary occlusion. Despite concerns that coronary artery occlusion on a beating heart would be associated with major haemodynamic instability and genesis of ventricular fibrillation, the majority of patients tolerate BHCAS well. Nonetheless, cardiac output may be dramatically lowered during the procedure due to compression of the heart, reduced contractility with beta blockade, heart displacement and ischaemia. There are two major components to the haemodynamic changes that occur:

• Manipulation of the heart.
• Ischaemia during coronary occlusion.

Manipulation of the heart

Preload optimization, together with careful slow handling of the heart, reduces the severity of haemodynamic compromise. The precise mechanism of the drop in pressure on lifting the heart is not clear, although it is probably the result of changes in right ventricular geometry and filling. For LAD grafting, the heart is lifted and rotated anteriorly with a swab placed behind it. This is generally well tolerated once the heart is positioned and appropriate volume loading undertaken. For right coronary artery/posterior descending artery grafts, the acute margin of the heart is lifted superiorly out of the pericardium and the effects of this can be ameliorated to some extent by placing the patient in the Trendelenberg position. Access to the circumflex vessels can be associated with abrupt falls in cardiac output. To minimize this, the surgeons may place deep pericardial sutures posterior to the left phrenic nerve and anterior to the pulmonary veins. Tension on these allows the apex to be lifted whilst maintaining left sided preload.

TOE can be a useful guide to optimize filling. Bradycardia, which may be desirable, can produce hypotension. Phenylephrine and noradrenaline have been used in combination with glycerol trinitrate to increase diastolic perfusion pressure and coronary blood flow. In practice, a combination of fluids and vasoconstrictors are used to optimize heart function during critical periods. Inotropes may be necessary.

Ischaemia during coronary occlusion

Superimposed on the effects of moving the heart is the response to coronary artery occlusion during anastomosis. Patients with stenoses of less than 80% without collaterals are at high risk of ischaemia during occlusion. This is brief, regional and resolves quickly once flow is restored. A study of coronary operations performed with and without

CPB showed superior preservation of ventricular function in the non-CPB group despite extended periods of unprotected regional ischaemia. Strategies have been sought to reduce regional ischaemia resulting from coronary occlusion during BHCAS. Attention has focused on ischaemic preconditioning, use of thoracic epidurals, intracoronary shunts and pharmacological agents.

The observation that a brief period of ischaemia confers relative protection against a subsequent more prolonged ischaemic insult has led to use of this approach (ischaemic preconditioning) during BHCAS. Brief occlusion of the target artery followed by reperfusion before grafting has been used, although no definitive benefit has been demonstrated.

Arrhythmias

Arrhythmias are undesirable during BHCAS because of associated falls in cardiac output or increases in ventricular rate which are poorly tolerated. The causes of arrhythmias are shown in Table 3.7.

Atrial fibrillation during occlusion of the right coronary artery may be resistant to treatment until perfusion is restored. Ischaemic arrhythmias that fail to respond may be an indication to convert to cardiopulmonary bypass. External defibrillator pads should be applied routinely to those patients in whom a limited-access approach is planned. Optimizing circulating potassium values and routine administration of magnesium reduces the likelihood of arrhythmias occurring intra- and postoperatively.

Haematological issues

There is no agreement about the degree of anticoagulation required for BHCAS. We administer 150–200 IU heparin/kg aiming for an activated clotting time (ACT) > 300 s, monitor the ACT every 30 min and give supplementaly doses of heparin as required. Other units employ

---

Table 3.7 Causes of arrhythmias during beating heart coronary artery surgery

Handling of the heart
Stabilizer attachment/detachment
Occlusion of the right coronary artery rendering the sinoatrial node ischaemic
Ischaemia
Reperfusion arrhythmias

full heparinization as for cardiopulmonary bypass. Protamine reversal is also an area of debate. Heparin neutralization may be unnecessary, and even undesirable, as patients undergoing BHCAS develop platelet activation postoperatively, leading to a hypercoagulable state similar to that seen after non-cardiac surgery. Most surgeons routinely prescribe low-molecular-weight heparin subcutaneously starting the day after surgery.

Early reports of MIDCAB showed reduced transfusion requirements compared with standard surgery.

Conversion to cardiopulmonary bypass

BHCAS is generally well tolerated, but it is occasionally necessary to convert the procedure to a more conventional approach using cardiopulmonary bypass. Conversion rates vary between units from 1% to 7%. Most surgeons agree that a perfusionist should be available for all BHCAS cases. Indications for conversion are shown in Table 3.8.

Postoperative period

Depending on the anaesthetic technique, patients undergoing MIDCAB and OPCAB procedures may be extubated in theatre, or shortly after arrival in a high dependency area. The absence of CPB alleviates problems of hypothermia, anaemia, electrolyte abnormalities and prolonged bleeding. One of the purported advantages of BHCAS is the reduced requirement for intensive care facilities and nursing postoperatively.

Ventricular function is better preserved in patients undergoing BHCAS and inotrope requirements are reduced. Patients with a thoracotomy have more pain in the first few days postoperatively than those who have had surgery with a sternotomy. Both epidural and intrathecal analgesic techniques have been used after BHCAS, but patient-controlled analgesia with morphine is widely used.

Table 3.8   Indications for conversion to cardiopulmonary bypass

Persistent ischaemia
Intractable arrhythmias
Uncontrollable hypotension
Poor access
Heavily calcified or intramyocardial vessels

Outcome

BHCAS appears to be safe, cost-effective and advantageous to patients in the short term. A 96.3% early anastomotic patency rate for LIMA to LAD via MIDCAB has been reported. Rates of perioperative myocardial infarction and death range from 0% to 4%.

The incidence of documented stroke after CABG surgery with CPB is approximately 3%, but more subtle neurological defects occur in more than 60% of patients. Although this is probably multifactorial, avoiding CPB should significantly reduce neurological injury.

Further reading

Ascione R, Lloyd C, Underwood M, Lotto A, Pitsis A, Angelini G. Economic outcome of Off-pump Coronary artery bypass surgery: A prospective randomised study. Ann Thorac Surg 1999;68:2237–2242.

Botero M, Lobato E Advances in non-invasive cardiac output monitoring: an update. J Cardiothorac Vasc Anaesth 2001;15:631–640.

Clements F, Shanewise J, eds. Minimally invasive cardiac and vascular surgical techniques. SCA monograph. Lippincott, Williams and Wilkins; 2001.

Janssen EW, Borst C, Lahpor J, Gründeman PF, Eefting FD, Nierich A, Robles de Medina EO, Bredée JJ. Coronary artery bypass grafting without cardiopulmonary bypass using the Octopus method results in the first 100 patients. J Thorac Cardiovasc Surg 1998;116:60–67.

Khan N, De Souza A, Pepper J. Off-pump coronary artery surgery – a review. Br J Cardiol 2001;8:459–465.

Koh TW, Carr-White GS, De Souza AD, Ferdinand FD, Pepper JR, Gibson DG. Intra-operative cardiac troponin T release and lactate during coronary artery surgery: comparison of beating heart with conventional coronary artery surgery with cardiopulmonary bypass. Heart 1999;81:495–500.

Lampa M, Ramsay J Anaesthetic implications of new surgical approaches to myocardial revascularisation. Curr Opin Anaesthesiol 1999;12:3–8.

Nierich AP, Diephuis J, Janssen EWL, Borst C, Knape JTA. Heart displacement during off-pump CABG – how well is it tolerated? Ann Thorac Surg 2000;70:466–472.

Mohr FW, Falk V, Diegler A, Walther T, Gummet JF, Bucerius J, Jacobs S, Autschbach R. Computer-enhanced 'robotic' cardiac surgery: experience in 148 patients. J Thorac Cardiovasc Surg 2001;121:842–853.

Octopus Study group. Early outcome off-pump versus on-pump coronary bypass surgery. Circulation 2001;104:1761–1766.

Reidel BJ. Ischaemic injury and its prevention. J Cardiothorac Vasc Anaesth 1998;12:20–27.

Anaesthesia for specific cardiac and allied operations

Coronary artery surgery

This procedure ranges from low-risk elective surgery, with a mortality of less than 1%, to very high-risk surgery in patients presenting as an emergency with poor ventricular function or significant comorbid disease.

The anaesthetist should make an assessment of the severity of the coronary artery disease before surgery so that the risk of intraoperative and, specifically, prebypass myocardial ischaemia may be quantified (Table 4.1). Preoperative assessment of the patient with ischaemic heart disease is discussed in Chapter 1.

Myocardial oxygen supply is directly related to arterial oxygen content and coronary blood flow which may be critical in patients with coronary artery disease. Myocardial oxygen demand is directly related to heart rate, myocardial contractility, wall tension (afterload) and myocardial temperature. The prevention of perioperative ischaemia in a patient undergoing coronary bypass surgery is dependent upon the optimization of myocardial oxygen supply and demand.

Table 4.1 Angiographic factors indicating an increased risk of perioperative ischaemia

- Left main stem disease: the left coronary artery divides to form the left anterior descending and the circumflex arteries, which in turn supply the majority of the left ventricle and interventricular septum
- Proximal left anterior descending and circumflex lesions: this amounts to left main stem disease
- Poor distal vessels: if the distal coronary arteries are small, or have diffuse disease, even following revascularization the flow of blood through the vessels will be low predisposing to early graft occlusion.

Most patients presenting for coronary artery bypass grafting (CABG) are taking drugs which affect these variables. (see Chapter 1). Beta adreroceptor blocking drugs reduce myocardial oxygen demand by slowing heart rate, and increasing diastolic perfusion time, thus improving subendocardial blood flow by controlling hypertension, and increasing myocardial oxygen supply. Calcium channel antagonists and nitrates increase coronary vasodilation, again increasing myocardial oxygen supply. These drugs must be continued until surgery, as abrupt withdrawal may result in rebound hypertension, tachycardia and loss of coronary vasodilation.

Patients with coronary artery disease often take aspirin which should be stopped 1 week before surgery in patients with stable angina to allow the production of a normal population of platelets. If the patient is at high risk for perioperative ischaemia and infarction, aspirin may be continued until the day of surgery.

Anaesthetic management of coronary artery disease

A thorough preoperative assessment by the anaesthetist is essential to fully explain the anaesthetic, answer any questions and allay any anxieties that the patient may have. Premedication is essential to minimize tachycardia and hypertension, temazepam is commonly used. It is occasionally necessary, in particularly anxious patients, to supplement this in the anaesthetic room with a small dose of intravenous midazolam, before arterial cannulation.

On arrival in the anaesthetic room, electrocardiogram (ECG) leads and a pulse oximetry probe are attached and peripheral venous access is gained. An arterial cannula is sited under local anaesthesia (with attention to whether a radial arterial graft is to be used). The patient is preoxygenated and anaesthesia induced with the principal aim of avoiding extremes of blood pressure and heart rate. A high dose opioid technique (e.g. fentanyl or remifentanil is commonly used (see Chapter 2). It is particularly important to prevent surges in blood pressure during tracheal intubation. Hypertension may be treated by increasing the dose of volatile or intravenous induction agent, or the administration of additional doses of fentanyl, midazolam, esmolol, metoprolol, or glyceryl trinitrate. Following tracheal intubation, whilst central venous access is being achieved, the blood pressure often gradually declines. If ventricular function is known to be good, hypotension may be corrected with the infusion of intravenous fluids. However, if hypotension is severe, or ventricular function is compromised, it is preferable to administer an alpha agonist, such as phenylephrine, to rapidly restore the diastolic pressure, and therefore coronary perfusion. Metaraminol, although commonly used in this situation, is less useful as it is mixed alpha and beta receptor agonist, potentially also increasing the heart rate and myocardial contractility.

Other surgical events that are associated with major haemodynamic changes, and therefore may predispose to ischaemia, include sternotomy, sternal retraction for internal mammary artery dissection, and peri- cardial and aortic dissection.

Despite adequate surgical revascularization, myocardial ischaemia is also common in the post bypass period. The incidence of perioperative myocardial infarction (variously quoted as 4.1% to 25%) is three times higher in patients who develop perioperative ischaemia. Furthermore, almost one-half of patients who suffer a perioperative infarct had either reinfarcted or died at the time of their 2-year follow-up, compared with 4% in patients who did not have a perioperative infarct.

Postoperative myocardial ischaemia may be due to native coronary artery spasm, or spasm in the arterial or even saphenous vein grafts, and is characterized by profound ST changes on the ECG, hypotension, ven- tricular dysfunction and myocardial irritability. Spasm appears to be associated particularly with the use of radial arterial grafts. It is therefore advisable to continue an infusion of a vasodilator, such as glyceryl trinitrate, into the postoperative period. Many surgeons also routinely use calcium channel antagonists in the perioperative and post- operative period to promote radial arterial dilation.

The fast track technique

Fast track cardiac surgery was developed in the 1990 as a method of maximizing the use of a limited number of intensive care beds. Fundamental to this technique is appropriate patient selection, exemplary surgery and the use of ultra short-acting anaesthetic agents, such as propofol, isoflurane and remifentanil (see Chapter 2).

Valve surgery

The perioperative mortality associated with valve replacement is currently 5.5% (UK Cardiac Surgical Register Data 1999–2000), which is substantially higher that that for CABG. This is in part related to abnormal loading of the ventricle and an increased incidence of asso- ciated myocardial dysfunction. Thus, in the management of these patients, the control of heart rate, preload and afterload in the prebypass period becomes particularly important (Table 4.2). All patients under- going valve surgery must have a preoperative echocardiogram

Table 4.2 Haemodynamic management before cardiopulmonary bypass in valvular heart disease

	Heart rate	Preload	Afterload
Aortic stenosis	60–80 beats/min Maintain sinus rhythm	Upper end of normal range	Avoid reduction
Aortic incompetence	80–100 beats/min	Normal range	Reduce stroke–volume ratio avoid diastolic hypotension
Mitral stenosis	60–80 beats/min Avoid atrial fibrillation	Upper end of normal range	Normal range, avoid increases in pulmonary vascular resistance
Mitral incompetence	80–100 beats/min	Normal range	Avoid increases in stroke–volume ratio

performed, and preferably all should have intraoperative transoesophageal echocardiography (TOE) monitoring.

Aortic valve disease
Aortic regurgitation

The clinical history in chronic aortic regurgitation may be misleading. Significant myocardial dysfunction may be present in the absence of symptoms. Conversely, sudden severe acute aortic regurgitation will result in signs of acute heart failure due to acute left ventricular diastolic overload.

The degree of left ventricular volume overload in aortic regurgitation is directly related to the size of the regurgitant jet and the diastolic time. Thus, premedication should be minimal to limit myocardial depression and promote a moderate tachycardia decreasing the diastolic time. During anaesthesia, a heart rate of 80–100 beats/min should be maintained, combined with an adequate preload to maintain forward flow and the use of vasodilators to produce a low systemic vascular resistance reducing the size of the regurgitant jet. This combination will reduce left ventricular distension, the size of the regurgitant fraction, and also improve subendocardial blood flow (subendocardial perfusion pressure = aortic pressure – end diastolic left ventricular pressure).

Aortic stenosis
In aortic stenosis, a heart rate of 60–80 beats/min is appropriate to lengthen the diastolic time, optimize myocardial oxygen supply and demand, and maintain the cardiac output. The blood pressure and systemic vascular resistance must be maintained within the normal range to preserve coronary filling during diastole. Although moderately raised filling pressures may be necessary to maintain the cardiac output, excessive infusion of intravenous fluids should be avoided as this predisposes to a rise in the left ventricular end-diastolic pressure and, consequently, a fall in subendocardial perfusion. The loss of sinus rhythm in the presence of aortic stenosis may have a disastrous effect on ventricular filling and must be treated rapidly.

Mitral valve disease
Mitral regurgitation
As with aortic regurgitation, chronic mitral regurgitation may be asymptomatic for a prolonged period. Pulmonary hypertension occurs late and the predominant symptoms, when present, are of a low cardiac output rather than pulmonary oedema. Conversely, acute mitral regurgitation will present with sudden biventricular failure as the left ventricle ejects into the normal sized left atrium causing a low cardiac output, pulmonary oedema and right ventricular strain.

The size of the regurgitant jet is dependent upon the size of the mitral valve orifice and the pressure gradient across it. In common with aortic regurgitation, premedication should be minimal. Under anaesthesia, to reduce the regurgitant fraction and maintain forward flow, preload should be maintained, a moderate tachycardia sustained and the systemic vascular resistance kept low. Most patients with longstanding mitral regurgitation have atrial fibrillation, this results in a loss of the atrial 'kick' to ventricular filling and therefore a higher heart rate is necessary to maintain the cardiac output. A pulmonary artery pressure catheter or a left atrial catheter (placed by the surgeon) may be a useful additional monitor of pulmonary artery pressure and left atrial filling following cardiopulmonary bypass (CPB).

Mitral stenosis
Mitral stenosis may be congenital or rheumatic in origin and usually presents with dyspnoea, often in association with pulmonary hypertension and right ventricular failure. The left ventricle is relatively under filled with a low-end diastolic volume and pressure. The marked dilatation of the left atrium almost inevitably results in atrial fibrillation, the onset of

which can result in a sudden severe fall in cardiac output and the associated rapid ventricular rate must be treated promptly.

Premedication must be effective as anxiety may precipitate a tachycardia. However, these patients are often small and susceptible to depressant drugs. A small dose of temazepam may be given 2 h preoperatively and, if necessary, supplemented in the anaesthetic room with small increments of intravenous midazolam. During induction, the heart rate should be maintained within the normal range (60–80 beats/min). Decreases in left atrial pressure (i.e. preload) and a bradycardia or tachycardia will considerably reduce left ventricular filling. Hypercarbia, hypoxia and acidosis will further increase pulmonary vascular resistance and must be avoided. Nitrous oxide, which is known to increase pulmonary vascular resistance, should not be used in the presence of pulmonary hypertension. A pulmonary artery catheter, or left atrial catheter, may again be useful in monitoring changes in pulmonary arterial and left atrial pressure following CPB.

Tricuspid valve disease

Diseases of the tricuspid valve are less common than those of the aortic or mitral valves. Tricuspid regurgitation is usually due to right heart dilatation secondary to pulmonary hypertension and mitral valve or, less commonly, aortic valve disease. Other causes of tricuspid regurgitation include endocarditis (characteristically in intravenous drug abusers) and congenital abnormalities. Generally, the nature of the associated mitral or aortic valve disease and the severity of the pulmonary hypertension determine the anaesthetic management, rather than the tricuspid valve disease itself, which is often entirely asymptomatic. Careful fluid management is essential, as in the presence of a dilated right ventricle hypovolaemia may result in a dramatic decrease in cardiac output. Conversely, over infusion of fluids may further compromise ventricular function. Unfortunately, the right atrial pressure is a poor indicator of volaemic status in the presence of tricuspid regurgitation, as the atrium and vena cavae are very compliant and a large change in volume may not be associated with any change in the recorded pressure. TOE is a useful monitor in this situation.

Returning to the general discussion about anaesthesia for valve surgery, following any intracardiac operation, air present in the cardiac chambers must be evacuated before the heart is allowed to eject. This may be achieved by manipulation of the heart and aspiration with a needle and syringe. Sites where air commonly collects include the left atrial appendage, the left atrial side of the interatrial septum, the apex of the left ventricle and the aortic root. The latter is particularly important as it predisposes to the entry of air into the right coronary artery which may provoke serious arrhythmias.

Following weaning from CPB, TOE is useful in assessing the adequacy of valve repair, prosthetic valve and ventricular function, and in the early diagnosis of a para-prosthetic leak. In the presence of long-standing valve disease, it is likely that ventricular function will be impaired and inotropes may be necessary in the early postoperative period.

Repeat cardiac surgery

The number of patients presenting for repeat cardiac surgery is progressively increasing as the morbidity and mortality from the initial operation continues to fall. Patients undergoing repeat cardiac surgery are at high risk, principally due to the progressive nature of cardiac disease, the potential need for more complex surgery, difficulties in achieving adequate myocardial protection, the increased risk of bleeding and the patient's advancing age and comorbid disease.

Anaesthetic management

The preoperative anaesthetic assessment should pay particular attention to the current status of the patient's cardiac condition, comorbid disease and any known perioperative complications at the time of previous surgery. Sufficient blood and blood products should be requested. Premedication is minimal and may be supplemented with intravenous midazolam, if necessary. The insertion of intravenous and intraarterial cannulae may be technically difficult, but must be undertaken before induction of anaesthesia.

The induction of anaesthesia should proceed with the utmost care. Following induction, the haemodynamic status of the patient must be maintained in accordance with their pre-existing disease, as described above. External defibrillation paddles should be applied, and appropriately cross-matched blood should be checked and made available in the operating theatre before incision as potentially catastrophic bleeding may occur on stenotomy. Drugs such as aprotinin or tranexamic acid, as well as platelets and fresh frozen plasma, may also be required in these patients to limit major perioperative bleeding. Intraoperative red cell salvage is a useful adjunct to further reduce the requirement for cross-matched blood.

Patients undergoing repeat cardiac surgery tend to have prolonged surgery. Effective myocardial preservation is more difficult to achieve, and the need for prolonged postoperative haemodynamic and ventilatory support is more likely.

Aortic surgery

Although not strictly cardiac surgery, surgery involving the ascending aorta and descending thoracic aorta is generally performed by cardiac surgeons. The ascending and thoracic descending aorta are principally affected by:

- Aortic dissection.
- Aortic aneurysm formation.
- Trauma (e.g. aortic transection).
- Congenital abnormalities (e.g. coarctation of the aorta).

The anaesthetic management of patients undergoing surgery of the aorta is at least in part determined by the site and extent of the lesion. There are specific anaesthetic considerations relating to the site of the surgery, as described below.

Ascending aortic surgery

- The arterial cannula should be sited in the left radial artery as the innominate artery may be cross-clamped during surgical repair.
- Surgery may include replacement of the aortic valve and reimplantation of the coronary arteries.

Aortic arch surgery

- Arterial access is usually obtained via the left radial artery and the femoral arteries.
- Cerebral protection is essential the management of deep hypothermic circulatory arrest is described in Chapter 5.
- Deep hypothermia is associated with a coagulopathy and bleeding may be severe.

Descending thoracic aortic surgery

- Surgery may be carried out without cardiopulmonary bypass via a left thoracotomy.
- A left-sided, double-lumen endobronchial tube should be placed to allow one-lung ventilation and minimize trauma to the left lung. Placement of a left endobronchial tube may be difficult in the presence of a large aortic aneurysm due to bronchial distortion.

- The arterial cannula should be placed in the right radial artery as the left subclavian artery may be clamped during the surgical repair.
- During coarctation repair, a femoral arterial cannula may also be used to assess any residual gradient.
- Descending thoracic aortic surgery is associated with a risk of paraplegia due to the potential interruption of the blood supply to the spinal cord. A significant degree of spinal cord protection may be gained by allowing the patient to cool to around 34°C.

Dissection of the aorta

Aortic dissection is classified by DeBakey (1955) into three types (Table 4.3) and by Daily (1970) into two types (Table 4.4).

Types I and II generally require emergency surgery, whereas patients with a type III dissection may often initially be managed conservatively.

Proximal lesions (i.e. DeBakey I and II and Daily A) may progress to involve the aortic valve annulus with resultant prolapse of the non-coronary cusp of the aortic valve into the left ventricle and severe aortic regurgitation.

Table 4.3   DeBakey classification of aortic dissection (1955)

- **Type I:** the intimal tear is situated in the ascending aorta and the dissection involves the ascending aorta, the aortic arch and the descending thoracic aorta: a proximal lesion.
- **Type II:** the intimal tear is situated in the ascending aorta and the dissection is limited to the ascending aorta: a proximal lesion.
- **Type III:** the intimal tear is situated in the descending aorta: a distal lesion.
    - **Type IIIA:** the dissection extends from the intimal tear proximally to involve the ascending aorta.
    - **Type IIIB:** the dissection is limited to the descending aorta.

Table 4.4   Daily classification of aortic dissection (1970)

- **Type A:** any involvement of the ascending aorta regardless of the site of the intimal tear: a proximal lesion.
- **Type B:** the dissection is limited to the descending aorta: a distal lesion.

Even with appropriate medical and surgical management, aortic dissection carries a very high mortality, particularly with proximal lesions. Rapid careful transfer of suspected cases to a cardiothoracic unit is essential.

Initial management

Patients with acute aortic dissection often have long standing hypertension, which coupled with the pain and anxiety associated with acute illness may result in an exceedingly high blood pressure. As extension of the dissection is promoted by hypertension, it is mandatory to rapidly control the blood pressure. Drugs such as glyceryl trinitrate, labetalol and sodium nitroprusside are appropriate.

As soon as the diagnosis is suspected (history, chest X-ray and depending upon local facilities, transthoracic echocardiography, computed tomography or magnetic resonance imaging), invasive venous and arterial monitoring must be established and the appropriate hypotensive agents commenced.

Once the patient has arrived in the cardiothoracic unit, the diagnosis may be confirmed with aortography in the catheter laboratories or TOE, preferably under general anaesthesia in theatre or on the intensive care unit. The passage of an echocardiography probe into the oesophagus, even in an anaesthetized patient, may provoke a profound haemodynamic response with severe hypertension and tachycardia.

Anaesthetic management

If an arterial line is not already *in situ*, this must be placed before induction of anaesthesia. Anaesthesia is then achieved with careful control of the blood pressure. If acute aortic regurgitation is suspected, afterload must be reduced and bradycardia avoided, as described above.

Additional vascular access must include at least two 14-gauge cannulae as blood loss may be excessive, in addition a femoral arterial line, a quadruple lumen catheter and pulmonary artery catheter should be placed within the central venous circulation.

Before sternotomy, the right groin is prepared or cannulated to allow rapid institution of cardiopulmonary bypass. In proximal lesions, the femoral artery is the preferred site for arterial cannulation as it is very easy to enter the false lumen if the ascending aorta is cannulated.

Surgery for aortic dissection is complex and may include the replacement of the ascending aorta, the aortic root including the replacement of the aortic valve and reimplantation of the coronary arteries, and replacement of the arch or descending thoracic aorta. If the dissection involves the aortic arch, deep hypothermic circulatory arrest is necessary to perform the anastomoses of the great vessels.

Aortic surgery may be associated with excessive perioperative blood loss. This is related to the complexity of the surgery and the coagulopathy secondary to deep hypothermia, if used. Cell salvage is recommended; however, the use of aprotinin remains controversial if the coronary arteries are to be reimplanted.

The continuing control of blood pressure is central to the postoperative management of these patients, as the entire false lumen is not usually resected during the surgical procedure.

Aortic aneurysm

The ascending aorta, arch and descending thoracic aorta may be affected by aneurysm formation usually due to extensive atherosclerotic disease. The surgical and anaesthetic management is dictated by the site and extent of the aneurysm.

Aortic transection

Aortic transection is a deceleration injury, usually sustained as a result of a road traffic or other high speed accident. As the aortic arch is fixed and the heart and descending thoracic aorta are relatively mobile, the tear usually occurs either in the ascending aorta or in the descending thoracic aorta just distal to the left subclavian artery.

The chest X-ray may be normal in almost 30% of patients who have an aortic transection, although widening of the mediastinum and loss of the normal aortic contour are commonly seen.

Echocardiography, or aortography, is used to confirm the presence, extent and site of the tear. The general principles of anaesthetic management are then similar to that for aortic dissection careful control of the blood pressure is essential.

Anaesthetic management

On arrival in the anaesthetic room, a right radial arterial cannula is sited to monitor the blood pressure during induction, surgery and, in particular, the upper body blood pressure during aortic cross-clamping. Following induction of anaesthesia, central venous catheters and a femoral arterial cannula are inserted.

During aortic cross-clamping, severe upper body hypertension must be prevented as the associated increase in afterload may provoke myocardial ischaemia and a deterioration in left ventricular function.

Conversely, upper body hypotension must also be avoided, as the blood flow via collateral vessels to the lower body may be inadequate to prevent damage to the spinal cord or kidneys. As well as normotension, mild hypothermia to 34°C may help to protect the spinal cord from damage during cross-clamping.

On removal of the cross-clamp, hypotension, and even rebound hypertension, may be troublesome. Blood pressure control is vital in the early postoperative period to maintain organ perfusion and prevent major bleeding from the anastomotic site.

Coarctation of the aorta
Coarctation of the aorta consists of a congenital narrowing of the aorta in the region of the ductus arteriosus distal to the left subclavian artery. The anaesthetic management is similar to that of aortic transection (see above).

Transplantation
Although some of the anaesthetic implications of heart, heart–lung and lung transplantation will be discussed; a detailed exposition of transplantation is beyond the scope of this book.

Anaesthetic management
The anaesthetist usually meets the transplant recipient for the first time in the middle of the night. Although this is not the ideal time, it is important that a thorough preoperative assessment is performed. Many of these patients are undergoing repeat surgery with implications for chest opening and the timing of the donor harvest and induction of anaesthesia. Generally, transplant patients do not receive premedication.

Upon arrival in the anaesthetic room, peripheral venous and arterial cannulae are inserted. Intravascular access and tracheal intubation should be performed under as aseptic conditions as possible because these patients will receive large doses of immunosuppressant drugs in the perioperative period. Broad spectrum antibiotics are given immediately postintubation. A quadruple lumen catheter and an 8-French sheath are inserted in the *left* internal jugular vein following intubation. This allows the preservation of the right internal jugular vein for post-transplant endomyocardial biopsies. Because the ejection fraction in these patients may be 15%, postinduction hypotension is common and must be treated aggressively with inotropes or vasoconstrictors. The administration of large amounts of fluid is inadvisable unless there are clear indications that the patient is hypovolaemic.

Heart transplant

Following implantation of the donor heart, with adequate myocardial preservation and the avoidance of an excessive donor organ ischaemic time, separation from CPB should be achieved relatively easily. If the ischaemic time of the donor organ is greater than 4 h, there is a progressive increase in operative mortality. Following implantation, reperfusion of the donor heart on bypass is allowed for a minimum of 20 min per hour of ischaemic time. Occasionally, the donor heart has pre-existing disease or has suffered an ischaemic insult which necessitates the use of inotropes or even a ventricular assist device. It is generally the right ventricle that fails due to an inability to cope with any increase in the pulmonary vascular resistance in the recipient. Post bypass, the heart rate is maintained at 90–100 beats/min as the denervated heart has an impaired ability to function adequately in the presence of an excessive preload. A useful pulmonary vasodilator in these patients is nitric oxide. A pulmonary artery catheter may be sited via the left internal jugular vein sheath post bypass.

Heart–lung transplantation

For heart–lung transplantation, a relatively large tracheal tube is used to facilitate fibreoptic bronchoscopy postoperatively to inspect the suture line. The tracheal tube is passed just beyond the vocal cords and the cuff inflated only enough to eliminate any leak of anaesthetic gases. The native and donor lungs may require repeated suctioning before and after the completion of the tracheal suture line, particularly in patients suffering from cystic fibrosis. The tracheal suture line and bronchial tree should be inspected bronchoscopically to confirm adequate clearance of secretions and the absence of major bleeding before separation from bypass. Inhaled nitric oxide is frequently beneficial in reducing the pulmonary vascular resistance in the donor lungs and should be immediately available in theatre.

Lung transplantation

Single-lung transplantation may be used in patients with non-infective lung disease (e.g. pulmonary fibrosis), whereas double-lung transplantation is indicated in the presence of infective disease (e.g. cystic fibrosis) due to potential soiling of the transplanted lung and the implications of immunosuppression in the presence of sepsis. Single-lung transplantation may be performed with one-lung ventilation via a double-lumen tube, whereas double-lung transplantation requires CPB unless performed sequentially. CPB must be immediately available in either case.

Excessive postoperative bleeding is a major cause of morbidity and mortality following heart, heart–lung or lung transplantation. This risk may be reduced by the use of aprotinin perioperatively and the timely and appropriate use of blood and blood products post bypass. The overall operative survival is steadily improving. Consequently, more transplant patients are presenting for non-cardiac surgery.

Further reading

DeBakey ME, Cooley DA, Creech O. Surgical Considerations of dissecting aneurysm of the aorta. Ann Surg 1955;142:586.

Daily PO, Trueblood HW, Stinson EB, et al. Management of acute aortic dissections. Ann Thorac Surg 1970;10:237.

Kaplan JA Cardiac anaesthesia London: WB Saunders; 1993.

Kirklin JW, Barratt-Boyes BG Cardiac surgery. Edinburgh: Churchill Livingstone; 1993.

5

Cardiopulmonary bypass

The first successful intracardiac operation to be carried out using a pump oxygenator was the closure of an atrial septal defect on 6 May 1953. Since that time, the complexity and safety of cardiopulmonary bypass (CPB) has improved almost beyond recognition.

Principles of cardiopulmonary bypass

The principal aim of CPB is to divert blood away from the heart via the right atrium or great veins, to oxygenate it, remove carbon dioxide and return it to the patient via the aorta to provide perfusion of the vital organs.

A typical CPB circuit consists of one or two venous cannulae inserted in the right atrium or vena cavae, a cardiotomy reservoir, a fresh gas supply with flowmeter and possibly access for an anaesthetic vaporizer, an oxygenator which may have an integral heat exchanger, a pump and an arterial cannula inserted into the ascending aorta (Fig. 5.1). In addition, there are suction devices, possibly a cardioplegia delivery system and haemofiltration circuit. The circuit also contains sampling ports, filters, bubble traps, and both pressure and temperature monitoring devices.

Cardiopulmonary bypass oxygenation systems

The blood is oxygenated via a membrane oxygenator as it passes through the extracorporeal circuit. The oxygenator consists of a blood phase separated from the fresh gas flow by a membrane. This membrane may allow gas exchange only by diffusion, or it may contain micropores of less than 1 μm in diameter, which allow direct mixing of the blood with the fresh gas for a short period of time after the start of CPB. The period of mixing is limited by the rapid deposition of plasma proteins on the membrane during the early phase of CPB, sealing the micropores.

The membrane used in these oxygenators is either in the form of hollow fibres or folded sheets of polypropylene. A heat exchanger is incorporated into the membrane oxygenator to allow accurate control of the patient's temperature.

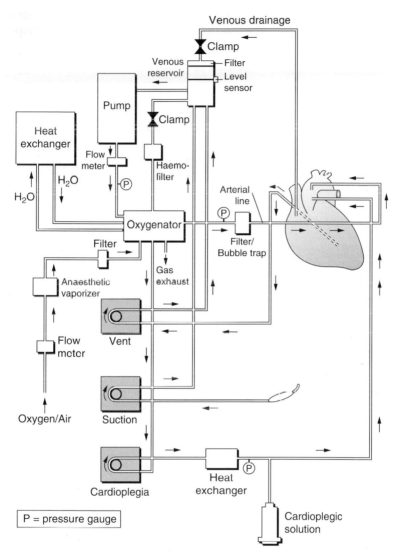

Figure 5.1 Schematic example of a cardiopulmonary bypass circuit. (After Gothard J, Kelleher A. Essentials of cardiac and thoracic anaesthesia. Oxford: Butterworth Heinemann; 1999, with permission.)

Cardiopulmonary bypass pump systems

Cardiopulmonary bypass pumps may generate flow principally via a roller pump or a centrifugal pump, and the flow produced may be continuous or pulsatile.

Roller pumps

- In this method of extracorporeal support, the blood is pushed through the tubing by a series of rollers.
- These rollers may be occlusive or non-occlusive, the degree of occlusion is often adjustable.
- Occlusive pumps may be associated with increased platelet activation and red cell damage unless carefully adjusted.

Centrifugal pumps

- Centrifugal pumps create flow either by a series of rotating cones or blades.
- This form of flow generation results in less platelet activation and red cell haemolysis than with roller pumps, particularly if the duration of CPB > 2 h.
- Centrifugal pumps may produce fewer gaseous and particulate microemboli.
- Centrifugal pumps are generally more expensive than roller pumps.

The flow generated by roller pumps may be pulsatile or non-pulsatile. In general, centrifugal pumps can only generate non-pulsatile flow. It is difficult to believe that there are no benefits of improved organ function associated with pulsatile flow, but this hypothesis remains unproven.

Filters in cardiopulmonary bypass

Macroemboli (> 200 μm diameter) and microemboli (< 60 μm diameter) are an inherent feature of CPB. It has been demonstrated that, although patients presenting for coronary artery surgery without CPB undergo some microembolization, the load is several orders of magnitude less than in those patient having the same procedure with CPB. Furthermore, the longer the period of CPB the greater the embolic load.

   Emboli may be:

- Particulate (e.g. atheromatous debris, clot).
- Liquid (e.g. lipid from the sternal bone marrow, silicone anti-foam from the bypass circuitry).
- Gaseous (e.g. micro bubbles within the bypass circuitry).

Emboli play a significant role in postoperative organ dysfunction and, in particular, brain injury. Much of this morbidity is caused by microemboli, in particular lipid microemboli released during sternotomy. It is important therefore to have filters in the bypass circuitry, particularly in the arterial line, to trap as many of these emboli as possible (Fig. 5.1).

Filters may also be used during priming of the bypass circuitry, in the cardiotomy reservoir, between the cardiotomy reservoir and the main circuit, in the fresh gas flow line, in the blood administration sets if blood is added to the priming solution and even in the cardioplegia delivery system.

The filters used may be:

• Depth filters, consist of packed wool or foam and have no definite pore size.
• Screen filters, consist of a woven sheet with a defined pore size of between 0.2–40 μm diameter.
• Micropore filters have a defined pore size of 5–40 μm.

These filters have been shown to reduce the risk of micro- and macroemboli passing to the patient, but they also contribute to the consumption of platelets during CPB. They may become blocked and a source of microemboli. Filters can also cause haemolysis and complement activation.

Vents in cardiopulmonary bypass

Venting the heart during CPB means the decompression of one or more chambers by a cannula, or designated suction catheter. This prevents distension of the ventricle and delays rewarming contributing to effective myocardial protection. The vent is attached to a roller pump and the blood aspirated is returned to the cardiotomy reservoir for reinfusion (Fig. 5.1).

Cardiopulmonary bypass priming solutions

Initially, whole blood was used to prime the bypass circuit and it was not until the early 1960s that crystalloid solutions were introduced. Crystalloid solutions result in significant haemodilution at the start of CPB, reducing the viscosity of the circulating fluid, so that organ perfusion is maintained even with profound hypothermia. This improvement in perfusion decreased post-CPB complications, including renal, pulmonary and neurological dysfunction.

Currently, 1.5–2.0 l of a crystalloid solution, such as Ringers lactate, is commonly used to prime an adult bypass circuit, to which 5000 units of heparin are usually added. A colloid solution, such as albumin or hetastarch, may also be added to raise the oncotic pressure of the prime and minimize postoperative oedema.

Drugs may be added to the priming solution in specific circumstances (e.g. calcium chloride, mannitol, aprotinin and corticosteroids).

In most patients, the inevitable haemodilution associated with CPB is corrected by a vigorous diuresis in the early postoperative period. However, in the presence of extreme haemodilution, a large circulating volume or poor renal function, haemofiltration may be necessary to avoid postoperative anaemia, oedema and increased organ dysfunction.

The pre-cardiopulmonary bypass period

The maintenance of adequate coronary perfusion with appropriate preload and afterload management is vital in the immediate prebypass period. There is often considerable haemodynamic instability, particularly during cannulation of the great vessels.

Heparinization regimen

Contact between blood and the artificial surface of the bypass circuit results in massive activation of the clotting and complement cascades; therefore, heparin is given to prevent potentially fatal coagulation at the start of CPB. Heparin is a highly sulphated polyanionic (negatively charged) mucopolysaccharide with a molecular weight between 3000–40 000 Da (approximate mean of 15 000). It acts principally by potentiating the activity of antithrombin III which inhibits the activity of thrombin and factors IXa, Xa, XIa and XIIa, thus inhibiting clot formation (Fig. 5.2).

Heparin is given in a dose of 300–400 U/kg via a central vein immediately before cannulation of the great vessels. The activated clotting time, measured from a radial arterial sample, rapidly reaches a plateau, confirming the action of heparin before CPB.

It is important that the heparin is given via a central vein (the lumen of the catheter should be aspirated first in order to confirm easy aspiration of blood).

The elimination half-life of heparin is variable because it is dependent upon many factors, including the dose given, the temperature and renal function of the patient. Regular assessments of heparin activity are carried out during CPB by means of the activated clotting time. An activated clotting time > 480, or three times the baseline value, is currently considered adequate to prevent coagulation during CPB.

Contact between the circulating blood and the surface of the bypass circuitry causes activation of the complement cascade, principally via

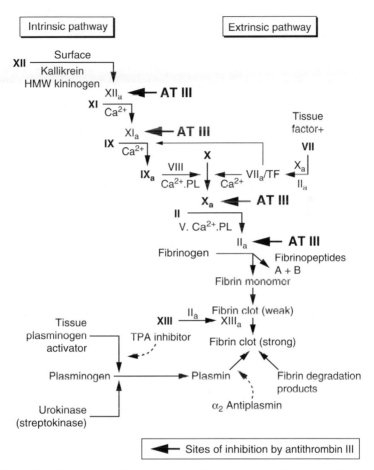

Figure 5.2   The coagulation pathway with particular reference to sites inhibited by antithrombin III (AT III). (After Gothard J, Kelleher A. Essentials of cardiac and thoracic anaesthesia. Oxford: Butterworth Heinemann; 1999, with permission.)

the alternative pathway. This results in cell lysis, vasodilation, histamine release, neutrophil and macrophage chemotaxis, and increased capillary permeability. It is this inflammatory reaction, in addition to macro- and microembolization, which is responsible for much of the organ damage that occurs post CPB.

Management of cardiopulmonary bypass
CPB is started by draining blood from the patient via the venous cannulae in the right atrium or vena cavae. The pump is started and the

blood and priming solution returned to the patient via the arterial cannula sited in the ascending aorta. The flow required during CPB is principally dependent upon the O_2 consumption of the patient. This is related to age, body surface area and temperature and is 4 ml/kg/min in the adult. A flow rate of 2.2–2.5 l/min/m² is adequate in normothermic adults.

The mean perfusion pressure during CPB is maintained between 50 and 70 mmHg. A minimum of 50 mmHg was established because it was easily attainable, it provided good operating conditions, it minimized the damage to blood elements on CPB, and was also the lower limit of cerebral blood flow autoregulation.

However, patients undergoing cardiac surgery are often older and sicker than the normal population and may have coexistent hypertension or cerebrovascular disease, necessitating a higher perfusion pressure.

The manipulation of the perfusion pressure may be achieved with vasoconstrictor and vasodilator drugs. Phenylephrine, methoxamine and metaraminol are commonly used to increase the perfusion pressure by their alpha agonist effects. If the perfusion pressure is too high, it is essential to confirm an adequate depth of anaesthesia and analgesia before using a vasodilator agent such as glyceryl trinitrate, sodium nitroprusside or phentolamine to reduce the perfusion pressure.

There is an immediate fall in systemic vascular resistance with the start of CPB. This is due to the reduction in viscosity of the circulating blood as a direct result of haemodilution and, according to the Hagen–Poiseuille equation, results in a fall in mean arterial pressure. This effect is generally transient and the reduction in perfusion pressure is usually short lived. The perfusion pressure gradually increases as CPB continues due to a progressive rise in systemic vascular resistance secondary to the extravascular absorption of the circulating fluid.

Other pressures monitored during CPB, including central venous pressure (CVP), left atrial pressure and pulmonary artery pressure should be maintained close to zero. In particular, any rise in CVP may indicate impaired venous drainage due to kinking or obstruction of the venous line, a malpositioned venous cannula or one of inadequate size, or an insufficient pressure drop between the patient and the venous reservoir. Impaired venous drainage compromises the perfusion of vital organs. It is vitally important that a raised CVP should not be assumed to be artefactual until all possibility of impaired venous drainage has been excluded.

Temperature management during cardiopulmonary bypass

Hypothermia is commonly used during CPB to reduce the oxygen requirements of the tissues, at a time when the perfusion of vital organs may be compromised. Blood and surface cooling are used to achieve the necessary reduction in core temperature:

- Mild hypothermia 33–35°C.
- Moderate hypothermia 28–32°C.
- Profound hypothermia 22–27°C.

A decrease in tissue oxygen consumption allows the utilization of lower flow rates, if necessary. The use of lower flow rates has several potential benefits. It may facilitate surgery, decrease the blood cellular damage due to the mechanical effects of the pump–oxygenator system, decrease the rate of myocardial rewarming via non-coronary collaterals improving the quality of the myocardial protection, and reduce the embolic load to vital organs.

Between 2°C and 5°C, cooling confers a significant neuroprotective effect in terms of reducing cerebral oxygen consumption and facilitating the use of lower flows. However, there is little difference in the incidence of cerebrovascular damage in patients who undergo CPB at normothermia or hypothermia. This may be explained by the notion that the three main mechanisms of cerebral ischaemic injury during CPB are thought to be macro- and microemboli, hypoperfusion and the inflammatory response.

Despite the obvious benefits of hypothermia, there are also significant disadvantages (Table 5.1). This has prompted the development of techniques involving normothermic CPB, which has been achieved without an apparent increase in morbidity or mortality.

Acid–base management during cardiopulmonary bypass

Dalton's law of partial pressures states that the solubility of a gas in a liquid is dependent upon the temperature. Thus, in the case of blood, CO_2 becomes more soluble as the temperature is reduced; therefore, its partial pressure decreases and the pH of the blood rises. During hypothermic CPB, two alternative blood-gas management strategies may be used, alpha stat or pH stat.

Alpha stat

The term alpha refers to the uncharged fraction of the imidazole group of histidine which provides the majority of the intracellular buffering capacity. During alpha stat acid–base management, although the total stores of carbon dioxide are maintained at a constant level, the pH, corrected for temperature, increases as the temperature decreases. Thus,

---

Table 5.1 Disadvantages of hypothermia during cardiopulmonary bypass

---

- Sludging of red blood cells if the degree of haemodilution is inadequate
- Complicates the interpretation of blood-gas analysis
- Drug metabolism is altered
- Impairs glucose metabolism with a tendency to hyperglycaemia
- Impaires coagulation and promotes heparin rebound
- Promotes electrolyte imbalance
- Cold agglutinins may be present which cause haemolysis
- Prolongs the duration of cardiopulmonary bypass predisposes to acidosis and postoperative shivering
- Rewarming may be uneven leading to regional ischaemia
- Predisposes to arrhythmias
- Causes gastric dilation, ileus, submucosal gastric erosions and haemorrhages
- Glomerular filtration is reduced, sodium, water and glucose resorption is impaired

---

blood managed with an alpha stat regimen is relatively alkalotic compared with that managed with a pH stat regimen. Under most circumstances, alpha stat management, which maintains a constant intracellular buffering capacity, is the preferred acid–base strategy.

pH stat

In pH stat management, as the partial pressure of CO_2 in the blood decreases with decreasing temperature according to Dalton's law, additional CO_2 is added to the blood via the oxygenator gas flows so that, when the blood gas is corrected for temperature, the pH remains in the range of 7.35–7.45 and the total body stores of carbon dioxide are increased.

pH stat management is principally used before and during a period of circulatory arrest as it improves cerebral blood flow by inducing cerebral vasodilation. This strategy allows the development of an intracellular acidosis; therefore, the period of pH stat cooling is often followed by alpha stat management which creates a relatively alkalotic state, helping to eliminate the acidosis and improve cerebral metabolic recovery.

Management of electrolytes during cardiopulmonary bypass.

The maintenance of circulating electrolytes, within the normal range during CPB, is essential. This is particularly important for potassium.

Factors predisposing to hypokalaemia during cardiopulmonary bypass include:

- Low pre-bypass potassium concentration especially in patients on intensive preoperative diuretic therapy.
- Hypothermia.
- The nature of the priming and cardioplegic solutions.
- Polyuria, particularly when mannitol is added to the priming solution.

Hypokalaemia should be corrected during CPB to achieve a serum potassium concentration of 4.5–5.0 mmol/l. Hyperkalaemia is less common but may occur if renal function is impaired, or multiple doses of potassium containing cardioplegia are used.

There is also a decrease in the ionized serum calcium and magnesium levels during CPB as a result of haemodilution. Although calcium salts are often given at the end of CPB, this is not only unnecessary, but it may also be deleterious as calcium has been implicated in reperfusion injury. Conversely, the fall in magnesium levels during CPB may be clinically significant and predispose towards post bypass cardiac arrhythmias. The administration of magnesium sulphate 2 g before terminating CPB may be beneficial.

The management of serum glucose is also important during cardiopulmonary bypass, particularly in the presence of normothermic CPB, cerebral hypoperfusion or if circulatory arrest is employed, because hyper- or hypoglycaemia have both been implicated in worsening ischaemia-related cerebral injury. The serum glucose concentration is maintained < 8 mmol/l for the duration of CPB. The administration of modest amounts of glucose post CPB may play a role in limiting reperfusion injury.

Anaesthesia during cardiopulmonary bypass

Adequate anaesthesia is essential during CPB to prevent awareness. Knowledge of the effects of CPB on the pharmacokinetics of the drugs used is crucial.

Anaesthesia may be maintained with a volatile agent such as isoflurane. The vaporizer is easily incorporated into the fresh gas flow of the bypass circuit and the expired vapour concentration may be monitored with a gas analyser attached to the waste gas port of the oxygenator. The blood isoflurane levels achieved by this method are somewhat lower than those found when isoflurane is inhaled. This may be due to differences in uptake of isoflurane from the bypass circuit compared with the uptake from the lungs.

Alternatively, an intravenous agent such as propofol may be used to maintain anaesthesia during CPB. This must be given via a central vein to ensure the reliability of administration. The concentration of propofol has been show to decrease exponentially with the duration of CPB because of sequestration by the circuit, although clinically this does not usually result in increased requirements.

It may also be necessary to supplement anaesthesia with additional increments of opioids and neuromuscular blocking agents during CPB. In particular, fentanyl is sequestered in the lungs and by the oxygenator membrane so that the plasma levels may decrease dramatically at the commencement of CPB. Subsequently, the half-life of fentanyl may be prolonged due to a reduction in hepatic perfusion during and post bypass. A newer potent opioid, remifentanil, also shows a significant reduction in metabolism during hypothermic CPB but, because its half-life is so short, accumulation does not occur and its duration of action remains predictable.

Cerebral function monitoring during cardiopulmonary bypass

Attempts to monitor cerebral function during CPB have been made since it first became apparent that bypass could be associated with post-operative neurological dysfunction. Traditionally, the electroencephalogram (EEG) was used, but this fell out of favour as different anaesthetic agents were found to produce different effects, and considerable expertise was required to interpret the results. Cerebral function monitors were then developed in which blocks of EEG data were subjected to Fourier analysis to provide trends in the fundamental frequencies. From these trends, information could be obtained during bypass about cerebral hypoxia and the depth of anaesthesia. More recently, the measurement of jugular venous oxygen saturation, auditory evoked potentials, transcranial Doppler and near infra-red spectroscopy have all been used (see Chapter 2).

Myocardial preservation

During CPB, a cross-clamp is usually applied to the aorta and the heart rendered ischaemic. Although this allows visualization of the surgical field, and facilitates a good technical result, without adequate myocardial protection, the period of ischaemia can lead to extensive and potentially irreversible cardiac damage. If the patient survives, the duration of hospital stay is likely to be prolonged and long-term recovery may be complicated by late onset myocardial fibrosis. The adequacy of myocardial protection is therefore of paramount importance to the success of the surgery. There are many techniques of myocardial protection available:

Crystalloid cardioplegia
Typical composition:

- Sodium 147 mmol/l.
- Potassium 20 mm/l.
- Magnesium 16 mmol/l.
- Calcium 2 mmol/l.
- Chloride 204 mmol/l.
- Procaine 1 mmol/l.

The advantages of cold crystalloid cardioplegia are shown in Table 5.2.

However, crystalloid cardioplegia does not prevent abnormal transmembrane ion fluxes, with the influx of calcium and chloride into the cells and the continued activity of energy-requiring calcium and sodium pumps. These contribute to depletion of ATP and the development of intracellular calcium overload, which is thought to be critical in the development of myocardial stunning.

Blood cardioplegia
Blood cardioplegia via the CPB circuit has emerged as the most commonly used protective strategy in the USA.

The advantages of blood cardioplegia are shown in Table 5.3.

A significant disadvantage of blood cardioplegia is that it is difficult to use with hypothermia because the increasing viscosity of blood at low temperatures limits myocardial perfusion. Warm blood cardioplegia has also been used, but has not gained wide acceptance.

Table 5.2   Advantages of cold crystalloid cardioplegia

- Hyperkalaemia causes the heart to arrest in diastole
- Multiple doses may be used
- Low viscosity
- May be combined with the cardioprotective effects of hypothermia

---

Table 5.3   Advantages of blood cardioplegia

- Improves oxygen carriage compared with crystalloid cardioplegia
- Improves buffering capacity compared with crystalloid cardioplegia
- Provides antioxidants to the myocardium
- Multiple doses may be used
- Warm blood cardioplegia may reduce reperfusion injury

Multiple doses of cardioplegia

Anatomically, all hearts have a significant, non-coronary, collateral blood flow. This progressively warms the heart and replaces the protective cardioplegic solution with systemic blood. These findings prompted the introduction of multidose cardioplegia and the topical application of iced solutions to the heart.

Anterograde versus retrograde cardioplegia

The protection conferred by any cardioplegic solution is dependent upon it reaching all the areas of the myocardium in a sufficient dose. Anterograde delivery may be by a cannula in the ascending aorta or directly into the coronary ostia. Effective delivery of cardioplegia via the ascending aorta is dependent upon a competent aortic valve, and the generation of an aortic root pressure of at least 60 mmHg to provide sufficient coronary flow. In coronary artery disease, it may not be possible to provide sufficient coronary flow with anterograde cardioplegia alone. Additional retrograde coronary perfusion with cardioplegia into the coronary sinus may, in these circumstances, provide more uniform myocardial protection.

Cross-clamp fibrillation

Intermittent aortic cross-clamping and induced ventricular fibrillation is not a method of myocardial protection; however, it may be used as an alternative to cardioplegia. Brief periods of ischaemia followed by reperfusion may reduce the risk of subsequent myocardial infarction in response to more prolonged periods of ischaemia. During surgery, this 'ischaemic preconditioning' occurs whilst the cross-clamp is applied to the aorta, ventricular fibrillation is induced, and the distal anastomosis performed. The heart is then defibrillated with a 10–30 J direct current shock and reperfusion is allowed to occur during the completion of the proximal anastomosis (Table 5.4).

Table 5.4   Advantages of cross-clamp fibrillation

- Allows the preservation of myocardial ATP values.
- Reduces the release of Troponin T (a biochemical marker of myocardial damage
- May be associated with improved postoperative ventricular function

---

In the presence of a severely diseased ascending aorta, the multiple applications of the cross clamp necessary to this technique may increase the risk of atheromatous macroemboli being released into the circulation.

Weaning from cardiopulmonary bypass

As surgery nears completion, the patient is rewarmed to a nasopharyngeal or oesophageal temperature of 35 36°C. If a peripheral temperature probe is also in use, the core–peripheral difference should be < 6°C. If rewarming before weaning from CPB is inadequate, significant further heat loss may occur while the chest is being closed. In turn, this causes shivering, increased peripheral resistance and increased oxygen consumption, all undesirable in the early postoperative period.

However, rewarming to a nasopharyngeal temperature > 36°C should also be avoided because it is potentially even more damaging than persistent hypothermia. The nasopharyngeal temperature upon rewarming consistently underestimates the jugular venous bulb temperature (i.e. brain temperature) by as much as 3°C. Thus, if the patient is rewarmed to above 36°C, as measured via the nasopharynx, the brain may be exposed to periods of significant hyperthermia, increasing the risk of neurological injury.

If an intracardiac procedure has been performed, one or more of the chambers of the heart are opened to the atmosphere and de-airing is necessary before separation from CPB (see Chapter 4).

The placement of temporary epicardial pacing wires may be necessary following bypass to protect against arrhythmias. Ventricular, atrial or sequential pacing may be used. Ventricular pacing is indicated in the presence of long-standing atrial fibrillation or if atrial activity is absent. Atrial pacing may be used in the presence of a bradycardia if atrioventricular conduction is intact, and sequential pacing is used if atrioventricular block is present. Finally, before weaning from CPB it is vital to correct any acid–base or electrolyte imbalance in particular hypo- or hyperkalaemia. Ventilation is recommenced and anaesthesia, analgesia and neuromuscular blockade must be reassessed and supplemented as necessary. All monitors should be functioning correctly and any necessary myocardial support instituted.

Separation from cardiopulmonary bypass

Once the patient is warm with a stable cardiac rhythm and all the above factors have been addressed, weaning from CPB may be started. The venous line is partially clamped and the heart allowed to fill. Then the pump speed is reduced to permit the heart to eject. If the blood pressure is maintained, the venous line is fully clamped. When the heart is appropriately filled and functioning well, the pump is stopped and weaning from CPB is complete. Subsequent filling of the heart may be continued by arterial line, if necessary.

The rate of weaning from bypass is dependent upon the adequacy of ventricular function. If ventricular function is poor, the period of partial bypass may be prolonged, whilst the degree of filling, heart rate and the use of inotropes are optimized.

The failing heart

Occasionally, despite careful preparation, weaning from CPB is unsuccessful, and without support the patient is unable to maintain an adequate cardiac output (Table 5.5).

As soon as it is apparent that the patient is unable to maintain an adequate cardiac output following bypass, the aetiology must be rapidly sought and appropriate therapy instituted. An objective assessment of haemodynamic status is necessary to guide treatment. A pulmonary artery flotation catheter may be useful, as may transoesophageal echocardiography. It may be necessary to reinstitute partial or full bypass whilst fluids, inotropes and other vasoactive infusions are commenced.

Table 5.5 Causes of failure to wean from cardiopulmonary bypass

- Poor preoperative ventricular function
- Inadequate myocardial protection
- Prolonged cross-clamp time
- Imperfect surgical repair
- Electrolyte imbalance
- Acidosis
- Arrhythmias

Inotropic support

Inotropic drugs improve ventricular performance at the expense of increasing myocardial oxygen consumption. As many inotropic drugs also affect the systemic and pulmonary vascular resistance, they are often used in conjunction with vasoactive agents, such as glyceryl trinitrate or noradrenaline (Table 5.6).

Mechanical support for the failing heart

Occasionally, even with optimal filling and appropriate inotropic therapy, ventricular function is insufficient to maintain an adequate circulation. Various devices are available to provide mechanical support for the failing heart.

Intra-aortic balloon counterpulsation

The intra-aortic balloon pump was introduced in 1962, and remains a popular method for treating cardiogenic shock, including that occurring after CPB. The device consists of a balloon-tipped catheter inserted via the femoral artery into the aorta, so that the tip is positioned just distal to the origin of the left subclavian artery (Fig. 5.3). The radial or

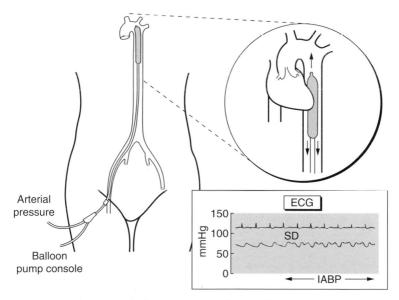

Figure 5.3 Intra-aortic balloon counterpulsation demonstrating the optimal position of the balloon, and the characteristics of the resulting arterial pressure tracing. (After Gothard J, Kelleher A. Essentials of cardiac and thoracic anaesthesia. Oxford: Butterworth Heinemann; 1999, with permission.)

Table 5.6 Inotropic and vasoactive drugs used commonly post cardiopulmonary bypass

Drug	Indication	Effects	Dose (µg/kg/min)
Adrenaline	Moderate to severe ventricular failure	Increased contractility, heart rate and systemic vascular resistance	0.01–0.6
Noradrenaline	Excessive systemic vasodilatation	Increased systemic vascular resistance	0.01–0.3
Dopamine	Mild to moderate ventricular failure, poor renal perfusion	Increased contractility, heart rate, splanchnic perfusion and systemic vascular resistance	3–10
Dobutamine	Mild to moderate ventricular failure	Increased contractility and heart rate, decreased systemic vascular resistance	5–20
Dopexamine	Moderate ventricular failure, poor renal perfusion	Increased contractility and heart rate, decreased systemic vascular resistance	0.5–6.0
Enoximone	Moderate to severe ventricular failure	Increased contractility, decreased systemic and pulmonary vascular resistance	5–20
Milrinone	Moderate to severe ventricular failure	Increased contractility, decreased systemic and pulmonary vascular resistance	0.35–0.75
Glyceryl trinitrate	Excessive pulmonary and systemic vasoconstriction, poor coronary perfusion	Increased coronary perfusion and venodilatation	0.1–10
Sodium nitroprusside	Excessive pulmonary and systemic vasoconstriction	Decreased systemic vascular resistance	0.5–10
Isoprenaline	Bradycardia and heart block	Increased heart rate, decreased systemic vascular resistance	0.01–0.1

brachial pulse should always be palpated in the left arm following placement to ensure that the tip of the balloon has not entered or occluded the subclavian artery.

The inflation of the balloon should be timed to occur at the dicrotic notch of the arterial pressure wave, which in turn corresponds with the peak of the T wave on the ECG (Fig. 5.3). Thus, inflation takes place during diastole and deflation during systole providing a wave of counter pulsation in the aorta. This counter pulsation increases the mean diastolic aortic pressure, which in turn improves organ blood flow, in particular coronary and cerebral perfusion. There is also a modest reduction in systolic arterial pressure, reducing the left ventricular afterload. The counter pulsation results in improvements in the myocardial oxygen supply, endocardial viability and cardiac output. Complications associated with the insertion of an intra-aortic balloon pump are shown in Table 5.7.

Reversal of heparin

Once separation from CPB has been successfully achieved, and the circulation is stable, it is necessary to reverse the effects of the residual circulating heparin. Currently, protamine sulphate, a sulphated polycationic peptide (highly positively charged) with a molecular weight of 4500 da is used. The dose is approximately 1 mg of protamine per 100 units of heparin given prebypass, or 0.8 mg of protamine per total dose of heparin given. A stable bond is formed between the positively charged protamine and the negatively charged heparin. Heparin is no longer able to bind to antithrombin III, and anticoagulation is reversed.

The severity of many of the adverse effects associated with protamine is related to the rate of infusion. Protamine should be administered over a period of at least 5 min (Table 5.8).

Table 5.7   Complications associated with insertion of an intra-aortic balloon pump

- Malposition
- Vascular damage
- Haemorrhage
- Thrombosis
- Infection
- Confusion
- Compartment syndrome

Table 5.8   Adverse effects of protamine

- Systemic vasodilation due to histamine and nitric oxide release
- Increased pulmonary vascular resistance and pulmonary hypertension in susceptible patients
- Impaired ventricular function
- Thrombocytopenia
- Leukopenia
- Fibrinolysis
- Anaphylaxis

Management of post bypass coagulopathy

CPB results in haemodilution of all the blood components. Platelet function and numbers may be further compromised by the effects of heparin, protamine and exposure to the abnormal surface of the bypass circuitry. Furthermore, if heparinization is inadequate, activation of the clotting cascade may occur and additional consumption of clotting factors will result. Careful attention to surgical haemostasis and the appropriate administration of protamine is generally all that is required to prevent excessive postoperative bleeding (Table 5.9).

Haematological management of postoperative bleeding

Transfusion of blood and blood products must be guided by local transfusion protocols and be targeted at specific abnormalities of coagulation demonstrated by a full blood count and clotting studies. The empirical administration of blood and blood products post bypass to prevent bleeding is unacceptable.

Table 5.9   Factors predisposing to bleeding post cardiopulmonary bypass

- Repeat surgery
- Known coagulopathy
- Ingestion of aspirin, warfarin or other anticoagulant drugs
- Local or systemic sepsis (e.g. bacterial endocarditis)
- Profound hypothermia
- Prolonged bypass time
- Inadequate heparinization
- Inadequate reversal of heparin
- Severe haemodilution
- Cyanotic congenital heart disease

Pharmacological management of postoperative bleeding
Following the administration of protamine, an assessment of the activated clotting time is performed. If this is prolonged and haemostasis is inadequate, an additional dose of protamine 50 mg may be given before further assessment of coagulation.

Further reading

Alkhulaifi AM. Preconditioning the human heart. Ann R Coll Surg Engl 1997;79:49–54.

Bannan S, Danby A, Cowan D, Ashraf S, Martin PG. Low heparinisation with heparin bonded bypass circuits: is it a safe strategy? Ann Thorac Surg 1997;63:663–668.

Bowles B, Lee JD, Dang CR, Taoka SN, Johnson EW, Low EM, Nekomoto K. Coronary artery bypass performed without the use of cardiopulmonary bypass is associated with reduced cerebral microemboli and improved clinical results. Chest 2001;119:25–30.

Buckberg GD. Update on current techniques of myocardial protection. Ann Thorac Surg 1995;60:805–814.

Christakis GT, Abel JG, Lichtenstein SV. Neurological outcomes and cardiopulmonary temperature: a clinical review. J Cardiac Surg 1995;10:475–480.

Gold JP, Charlson ME, Williams-Russo P, Szatrowski TP, Peterson JC, Pirraglia PA, Hartman GS, Yao FS, Hollenberg JP, Barbut D. Improvements of outcomes after coronary artery bypass: a randomised trial comparing intraoperative high vs low mean arterial pressure. J Thorac Cardiovasc Surg 1995;110:1302–1314.

Gravlee GP, Davis RF, Utley JR. Cardiopulmonary bypass: principles and practice. London: Williams and Wilkins; 1993.

Grocott HP, Newman MF, Croughwell ND, White WD, Reves JG. Continuous jugular venous versus nasopharyngeal temperature monitoring during hypothermic cardiopulmonary bypass for cardiac surgery. J Clin Anaesth 1997;9:312–316.

Hartman G. Pro-Con Debate: During Cardiopulmonary bypass for elective coronary artery bypass grafting, perfusion pressure should routinely be greater than 70 mmHg. J Cardiothoracic Vasc Anaesth 1998;12(3): 358–365.

Hett DA, Smith DC. A survey of priming solutions used for cardiopulmonary bypass. Perfusion 1994;9:19–22.

Kirklin JW, Barratt-Boyes BG. Cardiac surgery. New York Churchill Livingstone Inc.; 1993.

Nanas JN, Moulopoulos SD. Counterpulsation: historical background, technical improvements, haemodynamic and metabolic effects. Cardiology 1994;84:156–167.

6

The early postoperative management of patients undergoing cardiac surgery

Following completion of surgery, the patient is transferred to the intensive care or high dependency unit. This is a time of potential instability and the tendency by the theatre team to relax at the completion of surgery must be avoided (Table 6.1).

It is important to make careful preparations for transfer:

- The maximum available level of monitoring should be used.
- Infusion pumps should be checked for syringes that are almost empty and with limited battery life and replaced if necessary.
- The oxygen cylinder should be checked.
- Anaesthesia should be supplemented with further hypnotic agents and opiates as appropriate.
- Intravenous fluids should be primed.
- Vasoactive and anaesthetic drugs for bolus administration should be available.

It is not necessary to clamp the chest drains during transfer. Indeed, if they are clamped, it makes the detection of a sudden haemorrhage difficult and the patient may rapidly develop cardiac tamponade.

Table 6.1   Factors leading to destabilization during transfer

- Reduction in monitoring
- Hand ventilation of variable efficacy
- Infusion pumps accidentally switched off, disconnected or suffering power failure
- Short-acting anaesthetic drugs wearing off
- Continued rewarming leading to unexpected vasodilatation
- Continued bleeding leading to hypovolaemia

When the patient arrives on the intensive care unit, full monitoring and mechanical ventilation should be reinstituted as rapidly as possible and details of the operative procedure conveyed to the nurse and doctor involved in the subsequent care of the patient. A plan should be formulated, with the aim of early extubation, if appropriate.

During the early postoperative period, the minimum monitoring acceptable is an electrocardiogram (ECG) invasive arterial pressure and right atrial pressure, arterial oxygen saturation, urine output, chest tube drainage and core and peripheral temperature measurement.

Postoperative bleeding

Following closure of the chest, the chest drains are connected to an underwater seal and a vacuum of 5 kPa is applied. During transfer of the patient from theatre, the chest drain tubing is not clamped, but the bottles are transported at a level lower than the patient to avoid drainage of air and water into the pleural cavity. Patients undergoing cardiac surgery are at a significant risk of bleeding postoperatively.

Bleeding may be described as:

- Severe (> 400 ml/h).
- Heavy (200–400 ml/h).
- Moderate (< 200 ml/h).

It may be concealed, where it remains inside the chest as a pericardial or pleural effusion, or more commonly revealed, where it appears in the chest drains. Continuing haemorrhage may have a surgical cause, or be due to a haematological problem. Prolonged 'surgical' bleeding will inevitably lead to platelet and clotting factor depletion and an associated coagulopathy.

If the patient is bleeding moderately postoperatively, a minimum of 4 units of blood should be requested and a full blood count, coagulation screen, and a serum heparin concentration should be performed. If any of the tests of coagulation are abnormal, they should be corrected with infusion of the appropriate blood products.

Pharmacological management of postoperative bleeding (Table 6.2)

If bleeding continues or increases in the presence of a normal clotting screen, or signs of cardiac tamponade develop (increased filling pressure in the presence of systemic hypotension), the patient should be taken back to theatre and re-explored for a surgical source of the bleeding. Resternotomy under these circumstances is associated with an in-hospital mortality of approximately 20%. Occasionally, with severe bleeding, the chest may be reopened in the intensive care unit. Adequate analgesia, anaesthesia, antibiotics and muscle relaxation must provided for patients undergoing re-exploration under these circumstances.

The chest drains are removed on the first or second postoperative day, depending upon local policy. Despite the routine use of chest drains, the incidence of echocardiographic proven pericardial effusion following cardiac surgery varies between 26% and 85%.

Fluid replacement therapy

Following cardiopulmonary bypass (CPB), the extracellular fluid volume may increase by as much as 20% to 30% due to the volume of the priming solution given, haemodilution and capillary leakage. This extracellular fluid overload increases with the duration of cardio-pulmonary bypass (CPB). Coexistent with this extracellular fluid over-load, there may be a relative intravascular hypovolaemia. In the hours following surgery, the patient will continue to warm up peripherally resulting in increasing vasodilation, blood loss may be ongoing and the post bypass diuresis may be marked.

Moderate postoperative haemodilution, and the resulting reduction in viscosity, has been shown to increase coronary blood flow, cardiac output and decrease left ventricular work. A haemoglobin of 8 g/dl is well tolerated in otherwise healthy individuals undergoing cardiac surgery. Below this value, the benefits of reduced viscosity are lost as oxygen delivery to the myocardium is progressively compromised (Table 6.3).

Table 6.2   Drugs used to promote haemostasis

- Protamine: (1 mg/100 units initial heparin dose; 0.8 mg/100 units total heparin dose; 50 mg bolus postoperatively). Binds with heparin and prevents activation of antithrombin III
- Aprotinin: (high dose 4×10^6 kIU + 500 000 kIU/h; low dose 2×10^6 kIU). Serine protease inhibitor, preserves platelet function
- Tranexamic acid: (High dose 5 g; bolus 0.5–1 g postoperatively) Inhibits plasminogen activation and fibrinolysis
- Desmopressin: (0.4 μg/kg) Increases factor VIIIC and factor VIIIAg, promotes platelet aggregation
- Ethamsylate: (12.5 mg/kg) Improves platelet adhesion, increases capillary vascular wall resistance

Table 6.3   Fluid replacement therapy

- 1 ml/kg/h of crystalloid (e.g. dextrose saline)
- Colloid (gelatin, hetastarch) to replace blood and urinary losses and compensate for progressive warming and vasodilation
- Blood if the haemoglobin falls below 8 g/dl
- Platelets and clotting factors as indicated by clotting studies and full blood count

Postoperative management of serum electrolytes

- Sodium: major surgery causes as increase in the secretion of anti-diuretic hormone and aldosterone, resulting in water and sodium retention and potassium excretion. There is usually a decrease in serum sodium levels as the conservation of water predominates.
- Potassium: the renal excretion of potassium increases which, together with the diuresis that commonly occurs postoperatively and the long-term use of preoperative diuretic therapy, may result in severe post-operative hypokalaemia predisposing to potentially hazardous arrhythmias. Severe hypokalaemia may present as a metabolic alkalosis with ECG changes including ST depression, T wave inversion and marked U waves. The serum potassium should therefore be maintained between 4.5–5.0 mmol/1 by infusing potassium chloride 10–20 mmol in 50 ml of dextrose saline into a central vein over 30 min.

  Hyperkalaemia occasionally occurs postoperatively. A serum potassium > 7.0 mmol/l is associated with peaked T waves, atrioventricular block and broadening QRS complexes. This must be rapidly treated with calcium chloride 10 mmol intravenously and 50 ml 50% dextrose with 10 units of soluble insulin.

- Magnesium: hypomagnesaemia after CPB is generally well tolerated but, in high-risk patients, it may decrease the cardiac output, cause ventricular and supraventricular arrythmias and prolong ventilatory support. These adverse effects are treated by the intravenous infusion of 2 g of magnesium sulphate diluted in 50 ml 5% dextrose over 30 min.
- Calcium: serum calcium decreases following CPB. This is usually transient, and not clinically significant in adults.

Postoperative acid–base management

Disturbances in acid–base balance are common following cardiac surgery (Table 6.4).

If the lungs are ventilated, any disturbances of acid–base balance with a respiratory cause can be rapidly corrected by adjusting the minute ventilation. With a metabolic derangement, attention must be directed to treating the cause. A low cardiac output, hypovolaemia and poor peripheral perfusion are treated with intravenous fluids, inotropes and vasodilators. Hyperglycaemia and hypokalaemia should be corrected with insulin and potassium infusions, respectively, and renal failure managed with normovolaemia, diuretics and haemofiltration, as necessary.

Table 6.4   Causes of acid–base disturbance

- Metabolic acidosis: poor cardiac output, poor peripheral perfusion, impaired renal function, sepsis, hyperglycaemia
- Metabolic alkalosis: hypokalaemia, massive transfusion
- Respiratory acidosis: hypoventilation during transfer, inappropriate ventilator settings
- Respiratory alkalosis: hyperventilation during transfer, inappropriate ventilator settings

---

The management of arrhythmias following cardiac surgery

Arrhythmias following cardiac surgery require rapid and effective treatment (Table 6.5).

General factors such as hypotension, electrolyte imbalance, hypothermia and inadequate gas exchange, should be corrected before instituting specific therapy.

Table 6.5   Causes of postoperative cardiac arrhythmias

- Myocardial ischaemia
- Hypoxia
- Hypercarbia
- Surgical damage to the conducting system
- Electrolyte imbalance
- Pre-existing arrhythmia
- Drugs
- Pacemaker failure

Adverse rhythms may be controlled by physical or pharmacological methods.

Physical methods
Synchronized direct current cardioversion
Synchronized direct current cardioversion is a useful technique in the treatment of supraventricular tachycardia, ventricular tachycardia, atrial flutter and atrial fibrillation. A 50–360 J shock synchronized with the R wave of the ECG is delivered to the chest following correction of any predisposing factors, and induction of anaesthesia (Table 6.6).

Cardiac pacing
Cardiac pacing can be used to increase the heart rate in the presence of a bradycardia, or over pacing may be used to bring a tachycardia under control (Table 6.7). If possible, the sequential nature of atrial and ventricular contraction is maintained improving ventricular filling and atrioventricular valve function. This is best achieved with atrial or sequential pacing. The optimal paced heart rate must be determined for each patient but, generally, a rate of between 80 and 100 beats/min is appropriate.

Pharmacological methods
Commonly used anti-arhythmic drugs are shown in Table 6.8. Many postoperative cardiac patients will be receiving infusions of pro-arrhythmogenic drugs such as dopamine, or adrenaline. If an arrhythmia develops, rather than adding an anti-arrhythmic agent, a reassessment of the need for these drugs may be more appropriate.

Specific management of common postoperative arrhythmias
• Atrial flutter and atrial fibrillation

If hypotension is present, or the patient has signs of a low cardiac output, synchronized direct current (DC) cardioversion is the treatment

---

Table 6.6 Temporary pacemaker codes

Chamber(s) paced	Chamber(s) sensed	Response to sensing
0 = None	0 = None	0 = None
A = Atrium	A = Atrium	T = Triggered
V = Ventricle	V = Ventricle	I = Inhibited
D = Dual (atrium + ventricle)	D = Dual (atrium + ventricle)	Dual = Dual (triggered + inhibited)

Table 6.7 Common modes of cardiac pacing used in the early postoperative period

Mode	Function	Indications
VVI	Paces the ventricle Senses the ventricle Inhibits activity	Absence of organized atrial activity with intermittent atrioventricular block
VDD	Paces the ventricle Senses both chambers Inhibits and stimulates	Normal sinus node function with atrioventricular block
DDI	Paces both chambers Senses both chambers Inhibits	Sinus node dysfunction with intact atrioventricular conduction
DDD	Paces both chambers Senses both chambers Inhibits and stimulates	Normal sinus node function with compromised atrioventricular conduction
AAI	Paces the atrium Senses the atrium Inhibits the atrium	Sinus node dysfunction with normal atrioventricular conduction
AOO	Paces the atrium regardless of the intrinsic rhythm	The need for temporary atrial pacing in the presence of significant electromagnetic noise which may inappropriately inhibit the pacemaker

of choice. If the arrhythmia has been present for more than 48 h, the patient should be anticoagulated with heparin or warfarin to achieve an international normalized ratio > 2.0 before DC cardioversion to reduce the risk of embolization of clot from the left atrium. In the absence of heart failure, digoxin or amiodarone may be used to control the atrial rate.

- Supraventricular tachycardia

If hypotension is present, synchronized DC cardioversion is appropriate. Otherwise, vagal manoeuvres, such as carotid sinus massage or the valsalva manoeuvre, may restore sinus rhythm. If these fail, adenosine may be used. As adenosine has an extremely short half-life, it must be given by rapid intravenous injection flushed with normal saline. Other effective drugs include beta blockers, digoxin,

Table 6.8 Commonly used antiarrhythmic drugs following cardiopulmonary bypass

Drug	Class	Dose	Action	Comments
Lidocaine	I	1 mg/kg bolus dose 1–4 mg/min infusion	Membrane stabilizer, decreases $\dot{V}_{max}$, increases threshold, decreases rate of spontaneous depolarization	Negative inotrope
Esmolol	II	1 mg/kg bolus dose 50–200 μg/kg/min	Decreases rate of spontaneous depolarization, decreased sympathetic activity	Short $T_{1/2}$, cardioselective
Labetalol	II	5–50 mg bolus dose 15–120 mg/h	Decease rate of spontaneous depolarization, decreased sympathetic activity, alpha antagonist	Vasodilation
Amiodarone	III	300 mg bolus dose 900–1200 mg/24 h	Prolong the durat on of the action potential, increase refractory period	Long $T_{1/2}$, multiple side-effects
Verapamil	IV	5–15 mg in divided doses	Decreased calcium entry into the cells	Must not give with beta blockers
Digoxin	NA	0.5–1 mg in divided doses	Delays atrioventricular conduction, increased vagal activity	Toxicity is common
Adenosine	NA	3–12 mg rapid intravenous injection	Delays atrioventricular conduction	$T_{1/2}$ 8 s, contraindicated in cardiac transplantation

amiodarone and verapamil. Verapamil must not be given intravenously in a patient receiving beta blockers because it may cause
ventricular standstill.

- Ventricular tachycardia

  If hypotension is present, synchronized DC cardioversion is the treatment of choice. Otherwise, amiodarone or lignocaine may be used.

- Bradycardia

  All bradycardias can be treated with cardiac pacing, atropine or isoprenaline. Isoprenaline is contraindicated in patients with coronary
  artery disease because of the reduction in coronary perfusion secondary to the reduced diastolic pressure and increased heart rate.

Inotropic support following cardiac surgery

It is important, before starting an inotropic agent, to ensure that the
preload and afterload are optimized. In most patients, left ventricular
function determines overall cardiac performance; thus, assessment of
the left atrial pressure or the pulmonary capillary wedge pressure is
useful in the optimization of left ventricular filling. Transoesophageal
echocardiography is also helpful in assessing biventricular function and
volaemic status. If left ventricular function is impaired, afterload reduction may be beneficial before starting inotropic therapy. If preload and
afterload are optimized and the cardiac output remains inadequate, then
inotropic therapy should be commenced (see Chapter 5).

Dopamine

Dopamine has agonist action at alpha, beta and dopaminergic (DA)
receptors. At lower doses, its effect is predominantly at peripheral
DA1 and DA2 receptors causing vasodilation in the mesenteric circulation. In the kidney, DA1 stimulation results in renal vasodilation and
natriuresis, DA2 stimulation has a synergistic effect on the DA1 modu-
lated natriuresis. At higher doses of dopamine, the sympathomimetic
effects predominate with positive inotropic and chronotropic effects
via cardiac beta receptors, and vasoconstriction via peripheral alpha
receptors.

Dobutamine

Dobutamine is a synthetic beta agonist with predominantly beta 1 cardiac
effects. It has the disadvantage of causing a marked tachycardia.

Dopexamine
Dopexamine is structurally related to dopamine. It has marked agonist activity at beta 2 receptors and lesser activity at DA1, DA2 and beta 1 receptors. It reduces afterload via the beta 2 receptors, increases renal perfusion via the dopamine receptors and also has a mild indirect and direct inotropic effect. It has the disadvantage of potentially causing a tachycardia in association with vasodilation.

Adrenaline
Adrenaline is a potent inotrope with both alpha and beta adrenergic effects. The beta 1 effects result in an increase in heart rate and myocardial contractility. Its activity at alpha receptors also augments the blood pressure and decreases renal perfusion by causing peripheral vasoconstriction. Beta 2 receptor activity produces bronchodilation.

Noradrenaline
Noradrenaline has predominantly alpha effects resulting in peripheral vasoconstriction. It also has limited inotropic activity via cardiac beta 1 receptors.

Milrinone
Milrinone is a second generation type III phosphodiesterase inhibitor. It acts by increasing intracellular cyclic AMP which results in a positive inotropic effect in the heart and vasodilation in the periphery, including the pulmonary vasculature. Milrinone does not produce tolerance with prolonged use.

Renal support following cardiac surgery
Normal preoperative serum creatinine concentration does not preclude significant renal disease because the value only begins to rise when the creatinine clearance has fallen to less than 30 ml/min.

It is important to optimize renal function throughout the perioperative period. Factors predisposing to postoperative renal failure are shown in Table 6.9. Preoperatively, severe dehydration must be avoided. During CPB, the perfusion pressure should be maintained above 50 mmHg, and higher values are necessary in the presence of established renal failure, hypertension, peripheral vascular disease or diabetes. Postoperatively, attention should be directed at the maintenance of cardiac output, optimization of renal blood flow and the avoidance of nephrotoxic drugs.

Table 6.9   Factors predisposing to postoperative renal failure

- Preoperative renal impairment
- Diabetes
- Hypertension
- Hyperlipidaemia
- Complex surgery (e.g. simultaneous coronary artery bypass grafting plus valve surgery)
- Long duration of operation, cardiopulmonary bypass time, or cross-clamp time
- Red blood cell haemolysis or low perfusion pressure during CPB
- Poor cardiac output
- Increasing age

Nephroprotective drugs

Several drugs may be used perioperatively to help prevent renal damage. The maintenance of an adequate circulating volume and cardiac output are central to renal protection and attention should be paid to these factors before starting drug therapy.

Dopamine and dopexamine

As described above, dopamine induces renal vasodilation with a resultant diuresis and nariuresis. Although these effects aid fluid management, dopamine does not confer any specific protective effects upon the kidney. Dopexamine produces less renal vasodilation than dopamine. Both dopamine and dopexamine improve cardiac output, thus enhancing renal perfusion.

Frusemide

Frusemide is a powerful loop diuretic acting upon the loop of Henle to increase sodium and water excretion. Frusemide also has vasodilatory properties, increasing renal cortical blood flow and attenuating renal medullary hypoxia.

Mannitol

Mannitol is a complex carbohydrate, which is freely filtered by the kidney and acts as an osmotic diuretic. It decreases oedema of the renal tubular cells but, in excessive quantities, the osmotic diuresis may worsen medullary hypoxia. Mannitol also increases the circulating volume and decreases the haematocrit, both of which further improve renal perfusion.

Aminophylline

Aminophylline belongs to the xanthine group of drugs, it has mild inotropic and chronotropic effects and also causes peripheral vasodilation. Aminophylline acts as a weak diuretic by increasing the glomerular filtration rate and decreasing tubular reabsorbtion.

Urodilantin

Urodilantin is a polypeptide fragment of atrial naturetic peptide. It acts by dilating afferent renal arterioles and constricting efferent arterioles. This increases the pressure gradient across the glomeruli and promotes a diuresis and natriuresis.

Despite careful and appropriate management, up to 5% of patients develop acute renal failure post cardiac surgery and, of these, approximately 50% die.

Renal replacement therapy

The onset of acute postoperative renal failure is usually signalled by a period of oliguria: < 30 ml/h urine for more than 2 consecutive hours (Table 6.10). If sudden anuria occurs, the urinary catheter is usually blocked and a bladder washout should be performed. Once a blocked catheter has been excluded, attention should be given to ensuring that the cardiac output is adequate and that the patient is not hypovolaemic. If oliguria persists, despite appropriate fluid management and the addition of one or more of the drugs described above, haemofiltration or dialysis may be necessary to prevent fluid overload, hyperkalaemia, acidosis or uraemia. Haemofiltration is generally preferable in this situation because it is a less complex technique and patients are less likely to suffer haemodynamic instability secondary to major fluid shifts. It is important to ensure that all nephrotoxic drugs are stopped, nonsteroidal anti-inflamatory drugs must be avoided and aminoglycoside antibiotic toxicity prevented by closely monitoring plasma levels.

Table 6.10   Indications for renal replacement therapy

- Oliguria < 200 ml/12 h
- Fluid overload
- Potassium > 6.5 mmol/l
- Acidosis pH < 7.1
- Creatinine > 300 μmol/l
- Sodium > 160 mmol/l

Haemofiltration

Continuous arteriovenous haemofiltration was originally developed in the 1970s to treat refractory oedema; however, its application to acute renal failure was rapidly realized. The patient's blood pressure drives arterial blood through the haemofilter and then back to the patient through a venous line. The ultrafiltrate is collected separately and replaced with a suitable volume of isotonic fluid with an appropriate electrolyte composition. It is possible to remove 10–14 l of fluid per day using this method; however, the need for arterial access prompted the development of continuous venovenous filtration (CVVH).

CVVH is now the most commonly used method of haemofiltration in intensive care. It requires the insertion of a large bore double-lumen catheter. Blood is then propelled by means of a pump at a rate of 150–200 ml/min out of one lumen of the catheter, through the haemofilter and back to the patient via the other lumen.

However, both of these techniques of haemofiltration require anti-coagulation, skilled nursing staff and close monitoring. Complications include haemorrhage, inadequate solute clearance, haemodynamic imbalance, protein catabolism and inappropriate clearance of some drugs.

Weaning from mechanical ventilation

Following cardiac surgery, it is common to undergo a period of pulmonary ventilation. This may be as little as 1 h, or stretch into weeks (Table 6.11). Usually either synchronized intermittent mandatory ventilation with pressure support or biphasic positive airways pressure (BiPAP) is comfortable for the patient and allows early weaning and extubation, if appropriate.

Table 6.11   Factors leading to a delay in weaning from mechanical ventilation

- Pre-existing pulmonary disease
- Left ventricular failure
- Pneumonia or other systemic sepsis
- Neurological damage
- Electrolyte imbalance
- Pneumothorax, cardiac tamponade or pleural effusion
- Phrenic nerve injury associated with the use of topical slush
- Acute lung injury associated with cardiopulmonary bypass

If ventilation is prolonged for more than 10 days, percutaneous or open tracheostomy may be performed to reduce dead space ventilation, improve the comfort of the patient and facilitate weaning. When weaning is started, positive end-expiratory pressure is reduced, followed by the inspired oxygen concentration to 40% or less. Subsequently, the ventilatory rate is reduced until the patient is solely receiving pressure support ventilation. In many units, it is common for the patient to undergo a period of spontaneous ventilation via a T piece before extubation. This must be limited to less than 30 min because deleterious basal atelectasis will rapidly occur.

Acute lung injury following cardiopulmonary bypass

CPB inevitably causes a degree of acute lung injury, although this is usually mild and not clinically significant. It is probable that this deterioration in lung function is due to an inflammatory response caused by the exposure of the circulating blood to the non-physiological surface of the bypass circuitry.

Approximately 2% of patients suffer a severe injury and go on to develop acute respiratory distress syndrome (ARDS), which significantly delays their recovery. The lung injury is associated with a reduction in lung volume, a decrease in carbon monoxide transfer capacity, the loss of hypoxic pulmonary vasoconstriction and an increase in pulmonary vascular permeability. Together, these factors result in reduced pulmonary compliance, pulmonary oedema and deteriorating gas exchange.

Patients with acute lung injury require prolonged artifical ventilation and careful fluid management. Fortunately, the mortality from ARDS related to CPB is substantially lower than that associated with sepsis or any of the other major causes of the syndrome.

Postoperative analgesia

Although the pain arising from a median sternotomy is generally said to be less severe than that from a lateral thoracotomy, it may still be considerable. Other sites of pain include the site of conduit harvest (arm or leg), the pharynx, neck, back and groin, if femoral cannulation has been used. Factors known to increase the intensity of the pain associated with sternotomy include prolonged duration of operation, internal mammary artery harvest, milking and removal of the chest drains, and endotracheal suction. The pain is generally more intense in the first 3 days when opioid analgesia is required. This may be administered via the intravenous or epidural route. Effective acute pain management is essential, particularly during the first 24 h, to aid mobility.

Intravenous opioids are commonly prescribed following cardiac surgery, either as a continuous infusion or as patient-controlled analgesia.

Epidural analgesia is increasingly used to provide analgesia following cardiac surgery (Table 6.12). It remains highly controversial whether the benefits of epidural analgesia outweigh the risks. It is generally accepted that the epidural should be placed the day before surgery to aid the detection and appropriate management of any complications.

Postoperative care of the 'fast track' patient

'Fast track' cardiac surgery is the early extubation and rapid transit through the intensive care unit of suitable low risk patients (Table 6.13). For this to be possible, patient selection must be undertaken with care (see Chapter 1). The surgery must be well planned and technically excellent, the anaesthetic technique should include the use of volatile

---

Table 6.12 Advantages and disadvantages of epidural analgesia for cardiac surgery

Advantages	Disadvantages
Excellent analgesia	Full anticoagulation is necessary for cardiac surgery so the incidence of epidural haematoma is likely to be increased
Facilitates early extubation and improves early postoperative function	May predispose to bradycardia and hypotension
Vasodilates the coronary arteries and reduces the incidence of postoperative ischaemic events	Patient may be sedated for a prolonged period postoperatively making the detection of an epidural haematoma difficult
Reduces the inflammatory response to cardiac surgery	Difficult to schedule as the epidural should be sited several hours, or preferably the day, before surgery
Decreases the stress response to cardiac surgery	Has not been shown to improve outcome following cardiac surgery

anaesthetic agents or ultra short-acting drugs such as alfentanil or remifentanil and propofol. The intensive care or high dependency unit must be organized to facilitate early weaning and extubation. Of the patients deemed suitable for fast track cardiac surgery, early extubation is not possible in 10% to 20%. This may be due to prolonged CPB associated with surgical difficulties, bleeding, arrhythmias or poor ventricular performance necessitating postoperative inotropic or mechanical support.

On transfer to the intensive care unit following surgery, the anaesthetist should provide the intensive care team with details of the patient's preoperative characteristics, the anaesthetic technique, the operative findings and the post bypass requirement for vasoactive and inotropic infusions. It is generally accepted that the use of vasoactive infusions or dopamine up to a dose of 5 μg/kg/min should not preclude early extubation.

Synchronized intermittent mandatory ventilation or BiPAP is instituted and a propofol infusion commenced. If remifentanil was used in theatre and morphine has not yet been given, a bolus dose should be administered and an infusion commenced; remifentanil may then be discontinued. Continued rewarming is facilitated, if necessary, with a surface warming device. Gas exchange, acid–base balance and chest tube drainage are also monitored. The systolic blood pressure is controlled between 90 and 130 mmHg, deleterious arrhythmias are treated, and the patient is allowed to warm to a core temperature of around 36°C with a core–peripheral difference < 3°C. The blood gases and acid–base status are maintained within acceptable limits and the chest tube drainage should be less than 50–75 ml/h. When these preconditions are met, the propofol is stopped and the patient is allowed to wake up.

Once the patient is awake and able to obey commands, rapid weaning from ventilatory support occurs. Extubation is performed by

---

Table 6.13   Benefits of early extubation

- Improved cardiac function, in particular improved diastolic compliance
- More rapid return of mucociliary function
- Less atelectasis
- Reduced nosocomial pneumonia
- Improved patient comfort
- Possibly decreased costs

the nursing staff, when the patient is awake, able to communicate and comfortable. The respiratory rate should be within the normal range with a tidal volume sufficient to maintain adequate gas exchange.

This whole process is usually complete within 1–4 h.

Further reading

Cheung PY, Barrington KJ. Renal dopamine receptors: mechanisms of action and developmental aspects. Cardiovasc Res 1996;31:2–6.

Davis R, Whittington R. Aprotinin. A review of its pharmacology and therapeutic efficacy in reducing blood loss associated with cardiac surgery. Drugs 1995;49:954–983.

Fitton A, Benfield P. Dopexamine hydrochloride. A review of its pharmaco-dynamic and pharmacokinetic properties and therapeutic potential in acute cardiac insufficiency. Drugs 1990;39:308–330.

Llopart T, Lombardi R, Forsello M, Andrade R. Acute renal failure in open heart surgery. Renal Failure 1997;19:319–323.

Shipley JB, Tolman D, Hastillo A. Milrinone: basic and clinical pharmacology and acute and chronic management. Am J Med Sci 1996;311:286–291.

Shoemaker WC, Ayres SD, Grenvik A, Holbrook PR. Textbook of critical care. Philadelphia: WB Saunders; 2000.

Unsworth-White MJ, Herriot A, Valencia O, Poloniecki J, Smith EE, Murday AJ, Parker DJ, Treasure T. Resternotomy for bleeding after cardiac operation: a marker for increased morbidity and mortality. Ann Thorac Surg 1995;59:664–667.

7

Preoperative assessment of patients undergoing vascular surgery

Patients presenting for vascular surgery are similar to those undergoing coronary artery surgery in many respects. The population is often elderly with a significant incidence of comorbid disease, including hypertension, diabetes and renal impairment. Smoking-related respiratory disease is also widespread. Perioperative cardiac events are common as demonstrated by the 5% to 10% mortality associated with this type of surgery.

Assessment of patients undergoing vascular procedures is important because of the high incidence of perioperative complications.

The aims of preoperative assessment are to:

- Optimize cardiovascular, respiratory, renal and endocrinological status.
- Undertake further investigation where necessary.
- Estimate risk for individual patients.
- Plan the anaesthetic management.
- Arrange appropriate postoperative care.

Risk assessment

Attempts have been made to identify those patients at high risk of intra-operative cardiac events and develop approaches to optimize management and reduce risk. This has included multivariate risk factor analysis using clinical examination and routine tests and various non-invasive and invasive tests. Goldman et al. (1977) analysed data from 1001 patients to identify patients at risk of a life-threatening perioperative cardiac complication or death. They weighted various independent cardiac and patient factors to provide a score that estimates the risk of perioperative cardiac complications. Independent indicators included S3 gallop or raised jugular venous pressure, acute myocardial infarction within 6 months and abnormal cardiac rhythm. It was found to be in-accurate for patients undergoing vascular surgery. The Detsky Cardiac

Risk Index was an attempt to simplify matters and was applied prospectively to 455 patients, but was found to have a low specificity. In 1989, Eagle produced a risk index based on results of vascular surgery in 200 patients. A high score is classed as the presence of three or more of the following:

- Age over 70 years.
- Diabetes.
- Angina.
- Q waves on electrocardiogram.
- Ventricular arryhthmias.

If the results of dipyridamole-thallium scanning were added to this index, then greater specificity and sensitivity were achieved but only for patients at intermediate risk. None of the available scoring systems provide precise indications of the risk to an individual patient. However, high scores do indicate high risk.

History and examination
A detailed history and examination should be undertaken as usual. Specific questions should be directed to determine the nature and extent of the disease and any comorbidity.

Cardiovascular system
A clinical history of coronary artery disease (CAD) is associated with an increased incidence of postoperative myocardial ischaemia and cardiac morbidity. Many patients may be asymptomatic, with silent ischaemia, and hence difficult to assess. The presence of risk factors including diabetes, hypertension, age over 70 years, hypercholesterolaemia and smoking indicate that CAD is likely. Chronic stable angina represents a low risk, whereas unstable angina is a medical emergency and should be treated before surgery. Exercise tolerance may be difficult to assess because of claudication, and stroke may also limit exercise capacity. Two sets of guidelines address the issues of interventions to reduce the incidence of perioperative cardiac complications of non-cardiac surgery. The guidelines of the American College of Cardiology–American Heart Association were first published in 1996 and are being updated. The guidelines of the American College of Physicians support the use of preoperative testing and coronary therapies in high-risk patients who are undergoing major vascular surgery. These guidelines and numerous reviews conclude that coronary artery

bypass grafting or percutaneous transluminal coronary angioplasty should be limited to those patients who have a clearly defined need that is independent of the requirement for non-cardiac surgery.

In general, a detailed history and examination with standard investigations is sufficient. Occasionally, more sophisticated cardiological tests will be necessary, such as dobutamine stress echocardiography or dipyridamole-thallium scanning. An ambulatory electrocardiogram (ECG) may demonstrate silent ischaemia. Patients with refractory angina, or evidence of poor ventricular function, should be referred to a cardiologist for treatment. In most cases, this will involve pharmacological intervention and only occasionally will more invasive procedures be required. Angioplasty and intracoronary stenting are rarely required as part of the preoperative preparation of vascular surgical patients.

Patients with pulmonary oedema are at high risk and should be carefully assessed. Hypertension has not been clearly identified as a risk factor but diastolic blood pressure > 110 mmHg is associated with myocardial ischaemia, arrhythmias, neurological events and renal failure. The optimal period of therapy before surgery has not been defined and, in the elderly, treatment may cause more problems than the underlying disorder. Arrhythmias should be treated as appropriate.

Respiratory system

Emphysema and smoking-related lung disease is common. Patients should be encouraged to stop smoking preoperatively and physiotherapy and breathing exercises commenced 2–3 days before surgery. A chest radiograph should be performed routinely and lung function tests and arterial blood gases undertaken as indicated. Optimizing treatment with bronchodilators and steroids may improve respiratory function preoperatively.

Renal function

The development of renal failure is associated with a high mortality. Patients with vascular disease have renal impairment from a number of causes, including hypertension, diabetes and renal artery stenosis. The presence of abnormal renal function preoperatively is the highest risk factor for the development of renal failure. Renal function should be investigated preoperatively.

Diabetes

Diabetes is a primary risk factor for perioperative cardiac morbidity although many patients may be asymptomatic. Silent ischaemia is common. Autonomic neuropathy is associated with cardiovascular instability during surgery and sudden death can occur.

Preoperative investigations
Routine investigations include:

- Full blood count.
- Urea and electrolytes.
- Creatinine.
- Chest X-ray.
- 12 lead ECG.
- Clotting profile, if a regional technique is planned.

Further investigations should be undertaken as indicated by the history and examination. As a result of these investigations, it may be necessary to obtain specialist advice in relation to the cardiovascular, respiratory and renal systems. All cardiac medication should be continued until the day of surgery.

Optimization
Attempts to reduce morbidity and mortality, particularly in abdominal aortic aneurysm surgery, have focused on preoperative preparation as well as intraoperative strategies. The routine use of beta blockade has been shown to reduce mortality with the effect lasting for a long period after surgery. It has been recommended that, in the absence of contraindications, beta blocker therapy should be given to all patients at high risk for coronary events who are scheduled to undergo non-cardiac surgery.

High risk patients include:

- History of myocardial infarction.
- Angina.
- Heart failure.
- Diabetes.
- Inadequately controlled hypertension.
- Major surgery (i.e. vascular, thoracic, abdominal procedures).

Therapy is started days or weeks before surgery and the dose adjusted to maintain a resting heart rate of 60 beats/min. In an emergency, intravenous beta blockers can be administered perioperatively.

Other work has focussed on 'pre-optimization' with patients admitted preprocedure to a high-dependency unit (HDU) for insertion of a pulmonary artery catheter. Fluids and inotropes are used to modify the cardiovascular system and elevate oxygen delivery to predetermined goals before surgery. This has been shown to reduce mortality in selected groups.

Perioperative planning

There has been extensive debate about the benefits of regional anaesthesia versus general anaesthesia in high-risk patients undergoing noncardiac surgery. The choice of anaesthetic does not affect cardiac morbidity and mortality in patients undergoing peripheral vascular surgery.

Where the patient will be managed postoperatively should also be decided. Initially, most patients will benefit from a period in an HDU. Abdominal aneurysm surgery may be associated with significant blood loss and cardiovascular instability, which may warrant intensive care immediately following surgery.

Further reading

Boyd O, Grounds RM, Bennett ED. A randomized clinical trial of the effect of deliberate peri-operative increase in oxygen delivery on mortality in high risk surgical patients. JAMA 1993;270:2699–2707.

Mangano DT, Layung EL, Wallace A, Tateo I, for the Multicenter Study of Perioperative Ischemia Research Group. Effect of atenolol on mortality and cardiovascular morbidity after non-cardiac surgery. N Engl J Med 1996;335:1713–1720.

Cooperman M, Pflug B, Martin EW, Evans WE. Cardiovascular risk factors in patients with peripheral vascular disease. Surgery 1978;84:505–509.

Detsky AS, Abrams HB, Mclaughlin JR, Drucker JD, Sasson Z, Johnston N, Scott JG, Forbath N, Hilliard JR. Predicting cardiac complications in patients undergoing non-cardiac surgery. J Gen Intern Med 1986;1:211–219.

Eagle KA, Brundage BH, Chaitman BR, Ewy GA, Fleisher LA, Hertzer NR, Leppo JA, Ryan T, Schlant RC, Spencer WH III, Spittel JA Jr, Twiss RD, Ritchie JL, Cheitlin MD, Gardner TJ, Garson A Jr, Lewis RP, Gibbons RJ, O'Rourke RA, Ryan TJ. Guidelines for peri-operative cardiovascular evaluation for non-cardiac surgery: report of the American College of Cardiology/American Heart Association Task force on Practice Guidelines. Circulation 1996;93:1278–1317.

Eagle KA, Coley CM, Newel JB, Brewster DC, Darling RC, Strawss HW, Guiney TE, Boucher CA. Combining clinical and thallium data optimises pre-operative assessment of cardiac risk before major vascular surgery. Ann Intern Med 1989;110:859–866.

Fleisher L, Eagle K, Lowering risk in non-cardiac surgery. N Engl J Med 2001;345:1677–1682.

Goldmann L, Caldera DL, Nussbaum SR, Southwick FS, Krogstad D, Murray
B, Burke DS, O'Malley TA, Gorrol AH, Caplan CH, Nolan J, Carabello B,
Slater EE. Multifactorial index of cardiac risk in non-cardiac surgical pro-
cedures. New Engl J Med 1977;297:845–850.

Howell SJ, Sear Y, Yeates D, Goldacre M, Sear J, Foex P. Risk factors for
cardiovascular death after elective surgery under general anaesthesia. Br J
Anaesth 1998;80:14s–19s.

8

Anaesthesia for vascular surgery and postoperative care

The majority of vascular occlusive disease has been managed surgically but advances in interventional radiology have meant that many patients now undergo angioplasty or stent procedures under local anaesthesia. Both thoracic and abdominal aortic aneurysms have been treated with endovascular stents inserted via the femoral artery. The focus of this chapter is on anaesthesia for surgical procedures although the anaesthetist may be involved in some endovascular stent procedures requiring general anaesthesia. A brief description of these procedures will be given at the end of the chapter.

Patients undergoing vascular surgery are at high risk; vascular operations are prolonged and blood loss may be significant, and some patients will benefit from a postoperative period in an intensive care or high dependency unit.

Anaesthesia for vascular surgery

The aims of anaesthesia for vascular surgery are shown in Table 8.1. There are two main approaches, opioids supplemented with a volatile agent or a combined general and regional technique. Whilst opioids provide cardiovascular stability intraoperatively, their use may result in prolonged ventilation and hypertension postoperatively. Induction of anaesthesia is usually undertaken with short-acting opioids and an intravenous agent, together with a non-depolarizing muscle relaxant to facilitate intubation and ventilation. Maintenance may be provided by

---

Table 8.1 Aims of anaesthesia for vascular surgery

Maintenance of cardiovascular stability
Maintenance of circulating blood volume
Decrease in the stress response to surgery
Preservation of renal function

volatile agents or propofol by infusion. Longer-acting opioids may be given towards the end of surgery to provide postoperative pain control.

There has been extensive debate about the use of regional techniques alone, or in addition to a general anaesthesia, for vascular procedures. Epidural analgesia has a number of theoretical benefits (Table 8.2) and large series indicate that it is safe and reliable. If epidural analgesia is used for abdominal aortic aneurysm surgery, then thoracic insertion is necessary because the incision may extend up to the T6 dermatome.

If epidural analgesia is to be used for peripheral vascular surgery, the insertion of the epidural catheter should be the mid to high lumbar region. Both local anaesthetic agents alone, or in combination with opioids, may be used intraoperatively. Bupivacaine 0.25% is adequate if a combined general/regional technique is planned. Postoperatively an infusion of 0.1% bupivacaine with, or without, fentanyl or diamorphine is sufficient. The block should be achieved slowly with small incremental doses of local anaesthetic to avoid sudden haemodynamic changes. Preloading the circulation and judicious use of vasoconstrictors may be needed.

To reduce the risk of a spinal haematoma associated with anticoagulation, a minimum of 1 h should elapse between insertion of the catheter and administration of heparin. If thromboprophylaxis with low-molecular-weight heparin is undertaken, the epidural should be sited not less than 2 h before or 12 h after heparin administration.

Monitoring

Both non-invasive and invasive monitoring should be started before induction of anaesthesia. Non-invasive monitoring requirements are similar to those for cardiac surgery (see Chapter 2).

Table 8.2   Reported benefits of regional anaesthesia for vascular surgery

Attenuation of the stress response to surgery
Improvement in myocardial oxygen supply/demand balance
Cardiovascular stability
Attenuation of the response to aortic cross clamping
Improved endocardial blood flow
Reduction in requirement for general anaesthetic agents, particularly opioids
Improved graft and lower extremity blood flow
Excellent postoperative analgesia
Preservation of pulmonary function

Cardiovascular

Intra-arterial pressure measurement is mandatory as changes may occur rapidly with aortic cross-clamping or major blood loss. Central venous access allows assessment of right-sided filling pressure and the administration of inotropes, if necessary. The use of pulmonary artery flotation catheters is debatable and benefits have not been clearly demonstrated during vascular surgery. Transoesophageal echocardiography is used increasingly. It is relatively non-invasive and provides real-time information about filling status, myocardial function and ischaemia; however, it requires an experienced operator and is expensive.

Temperature

Monitoring of central and peripheral temperature is advisable. The aim is to maintain normothermia using forced air warming devices and fluid warming systems. Despite theoretical benefits from mild hypothermia, such as brain and spinal cord protection, it is associated with vasoconstriction and increased myocardial oxygen demand. Areas below the clamp site should not be actively warmed.

Haematology

Heparin is given before arterial clamping. Usually a single bolus of 3–5000 IU is given to keep the activated clotting time > 200 s for the duration of arterial occlusion. Protamine reversal is not usually necessary, any residual heparinization is beneficial for graft patency. Estimation of blood loss can be difficult. Routine haemoglobin or haematocrit measurement from blood gas analysis is helpful and a low haematocrit (< 28%) may be associated with myocardial ischaemia in vascular surgical patients. Appropriate venous access with wide bore peripheral, or centrally placed, cannulae facilitates rapid transfusion. The need for homologous blood can be reduced by techniques discussed earlier (see Chapter 5).

Coagulation abnormalities can result from gut ischaemia or excessive blood loss, and fibrinolysis may occur in supracoeliac cases. Laboratory tests are needed to characterize and guide appropriate management of the coagulopathy.

Renal function

Renal impairment is common and perioperative renal failure has a mortality of up to 25%. The key to preservation of renal function during aortic surgery is to maintain circulating volume and cardiac output whilst monitoring urine output. Suprarenal cross-clamping reduces renal blood flow and is associated with a higher incidence of renal

---

Table 8.3   Strategies to enhance spinal cord protection

Minimize cross-clamp time
Preserve critical vessels during surgery

---

failure. As in cardiac procedures, the use of low dose dopamine, loop diuretics and mannitol is common, but none has been shown to prevent acute renal failure.

Spinal cord monitoring

Spinal cord damage is a rare but catastrophic complication of aortic surgery. The main artery supplying the spinal cord is the artery of Adamkiewicz, which can arise anywhere between T1 and L1. Occlusion of this vessel results in spinal cord ischaemia leading to flaccid paralysis. Strategies for reducing the likelihood of spinal cord damage are shown in Table 8.3.

Cross-clamp application

The physiological effects of this manoeuvre depend on a number of factors shown in Table 8.4. The cardiovascular effects are dependent on how proximally the clamp is positioned. The potential cardiovascular effects of cross clamping are shown in Table 8.5.

Table 8.4   Factors affecting response to cross-clamp application

---

Preoperative myocardial function
Site of clamp application
Aortic pathology
Volume status
Anaesthetic technique

Table 8.5   Cardiovascular effects of cross-clamp application

---

Rise in systemic vascular resistance and afterload
Increased left ventricular end-systolic pressure and wall tension
Reduced ejection fraction
Fall in cardiac index and stroke volume (up to 40%)
Reduced subendocardial blood flow
Myocardial ischaemia with reduced contractility, in susceptible patients

Patients with normal myocardial function usually tolerate these changes well providing they are not hypovolaemic. Patients with ischaemic heart disease may develop ischaemia with reduced contractility, cardiac failure and arrhythmias. Blood flow to the gut and kidneys are reduced if suprarenal or supracoeliac clamping is required. Intravascular filling should be optimized before clamp placement and afterload reduced with intravenous nitrates or increased depth of anaesthesia. Inotropes may be required if these interventions are not effective in restoring cardiac output.

During the period of ischaemia, anaerobic metabolism occurs distal to the clamp with vasodilation. On reperfusion, hypotension occurs due to a sudden reduction in afterload, washout of anaerobic metabolites and lactate from the lower limbs and, possibly, reduced myocardial function in response to acidosis and a decrease in coronary blood flow. Adequate filling before clamp removal with slow release of the cross-clamp attenuates these effects. The distal clamps should be released first with each leg reperfused in turn.

Vasoconstrictors and inotropes may be required during this period.

Fluid management may be complex. Depending on the duration and extent of surgery, there will be significant third space losses and fluid shifts, particularly into the gut and retroperitoneal space. Hypovolaemia is poorly tolerated if a regional block has been used, and excessive fluid may produce cardiac failure in patients with poor ventricular function. Meticulous attention to variables such as haemodynamics, central venous pressure, urine output and acid–base balance facilitates the rational use of intravenous fluids.

Abdominal aortic aneurysm surgery

A recent UK audit of non-emergency infrarenal aortic surgery found an overall mortality of 7.3%. Factors associated with an increased risk of death are shown in Table 8.6. For emergency aneurysm surgery,

---

Table 8.6 Factors associated with increased mortality in infrarenal aortic aneurysm surgery

Age > 74 years
Urgent surgery
Operation for occlusive disease
Limited exercise capacity
History of severe angina or cardiac failure
Presence of ventricular ectopics

mortality around 50% is common. Aneurysms greater than 6 cm diameter carry an annual risk of rupture of 25% but no advantage from the early repair of smaller aneurysms has been demonstrated.

Management of ruptured aortic aneurysms

Bleeding, or imminent rupture, of an abdominal aortic aneurysm is a surgical emergency. There is little time for preoperative preparation and investigation, and surgery should be undertaken as soon as possible. The urgent cross-matching of at least 6 units of blood is mandatory. Preinduction resuscitation is the subject of much debate. On the one hand, the patient is suffering from haemorrhagic shock and it would seem sensible to administer fluids rapidly; however, aggressive fluid management may raise blood pressure, dislodge clot and result in further haemorrhage. Despite this, fluids should be given to patients showing signs of myocardial or cerebral ischaemia. Anaesthesia should be induced after good venous access has been established and a range of drugs including vasopressors and adrenaline should be prepared. Invasive arterial monitoring and central venous access are highly desirable, but not essential.

After a rapid sequence induction, surgery starts. A potent short-acting opioid, such as alfentanil, attenuates the pressor response to intubation which may cause further haemorrhage. This is a time of major haemodynamic instability and, profound hypotension, and cardiac arrest can occur. Rapid infusion of fluid may be required with the administration of vasoconstrictors. The aim is to maintain adequate perfusion of vital organs until the cross-clamp can be applied, first to the neck of the aneurysm and then to the iliac arteries. Once this is achieved, some degree of cardiovascular stability can be restored; indeed, hypertension may occur which can be controlled using intravenous glyceryl trinitrate and/or deepening anaesthesia.

Central venous access is obtained during the period of cross-clamping. If not already in place. A nasogastric tube is inserted and any other monitoring such as peripheral and central temperature, instituted. Arterial blood gas analysis indicates the severity of the acidosis and anaemia. Whilst the former may not be corrected until adequate perfusion is restored, the latter should be treated to maintain a haemoglobin of 9–10 g/dl. Coagulopathy is common due to haemodilution and release of thromboplastins from the ruptured aneurysm. Fresh frozen plasma and platelet concentrates should be ordered at the earliest opportunity and empirical treatment of bleeding undertaken until clotting studies are available. Renal perfusion may be severely compromised as a result of a low cardiac output and correction of hypovolaemia is the most important measure is preventing acute renal failure. Cross-clamp release should be undertaken in the same manner as described for elective aneurysm surgery.

Laparoscopically assisted abdominal aortic aneurysm repair

Much of the mortality associated with conventional repair of abdominal aortic aneurysms relates to the large abdominal incision, retroperitoneal dissection, bowel manipulation, blood loss and hypothermia-induced coagulopathy. A laparoscopic approach combines a less invasive technique with a conventional repair. This approach is demanding but early results are promising with low blood loss, on-table extubation and rapid recovery.

Peripheral vascular surgery

Perioperative mortality for peripheral limb revascularization is 2% to 6%. This increases with age and more distal surgery. Some patients are suitable for interventional radiological procedures.

The advantages and disadvantages of regional and general anaesthesia for peripheral vascular surgery are shown in Table 8.7. Despite

Table 8.7   Comparison of local and general anaesthesia for peripheral vascular surgery

Technique	Advantages	Disadvantages
General	Reliable	Variable postoperative analgesia
	Cardiovascular control	Postoperative hypertension
	Good patient tolerance	Respiratory complications
	Variety of techniques	Postoperative nausea and vomiting with opioids
		Hypercoagulable state postoperatively
Regional	Reduced stress response	Technical difficulties
	Improved graft flow	Patient may refuse
	Preserved respiratory function	May cause hypotension
	Reduced venous thrombosis	Risk of haematoma/nerve injuries
	Beneficial cardiac effects	

theoretical benefits of regional techniques, these do not affect outcome in terms of cardiovascular complications or death.

Whichever technique is selected, monitoring should be commenced before induction of anaesthesia or insertion of the epidural catheter. This must include invasive arterial monitoring and central venous access. Regional anaesthesia accentuates the response to hypovolaemia and hypotension may occur suddenly. If sedation is used in patients with marginal respiratory function, then regular arterial blood gas monitoring is essential.

Acute limb ischaemia

Acute limb ischaemia results from thrombosis or embolism and results in a painful white, pulseless limb. Thrombosis may be treated with intra-arterial thrombolytic agents, such as urokinase, alteplase or reteplase, which are a less invasive means of restoring perfusion. Embolic causes of acute ischaemia require urgent surgery using a Fogarty balloon embolectomy catheter. Embolectomy can be performed using local anaesthetic infiltration. However, many of these patients require haemodynamic monitoring, fluid resuscitation and systemic analgesia. Sedation can be used if the patient is monitored appropriately. Regional blocks may be suitable, but are contraindicated if thrombolytic drugs have been used, and may mask the signs of compartment syndrome. A light general anaesthetic is probably the most sensible option.

Amputation

If revascularization fails, then lower limb amputation may be necessary. It may also be required for chronic sepsis or intractable pain. Amputation has a significant morbidity and mortality and represents the end of a long and debilitating illness. Amputation is rarely an emergency and careful preoperative assessment and optimization should be undertaken. These patients are often very high risk with extensive comorbidity. Whilst either general or regional anaesthesia may be used, unilateral spinal provides excellent analgesia with minimal cardiovascular effects. Perineural catheters can be placed at the time of surgery into the sciatic nerve sheath for above knee amputation or near the anterior–tibial nerve for below knee amputation. These patients require meticulous perioperative management.

Phantom limb complex occurs in up to 75% of amputees postoperatively and may be a persistent problem for a significant number of patients. There are three elements to the phantom complex:

- Phantom limb pain: painful sensations referred to the absent limb.
- Phantom limb sensation: any sensation, other than pain, in the absent limb.
- Stump pain: pain localized in the stump.

The occurrence of phantom pain is independent of age, gender and level or side of amputation. It commonly arises early in the postoperative period, is intermittent and localized to the distal parts of the affected limb. It is more likely if chronic pain was a problem before surgery. Phantom sensation is almost universal in amputees but is rarely a problem. Stump pain usually subsides with healing. It has been suggested that regional techniques may reduce the likelihood of a patient developing phantom limb pain but this has not been conclusively demonstrated. Whatever technique is used, effective, analgesia is essential both pre- and postoperatively.

Upper limb surgery
Vascular procedures are rarely required on the arm, although acute ischaemia can result from an embolus, usually from the heart, and surgery may be required following trauma.

Postoperative care
Following abdominal aortic aneurysm surgery, patients have traditionally been admitted to an intensive care unit for the reasons shown in Table 8.8. After emergency aortic aneurysm repair all these factors are present and admission to the intensive care unit is mandatory. However, after elective aortic or peripheral vascular surgery, transfer to a high-dependency unit (HDU) may be appropriate. 'Fast-tracking' of selected patients has been used to reduce the need for intensive care beds. The

---

Table 8.8   Reasons for admission to intensive care unit after vascular surgery

Prolonged/emergency surgery
Elderly patients
Massive blood loss
Cardiovascular instability
Persistent acidosis
Poor respiratory reserve requiring post-operative ventilation
Use of epidural analgesia

increased use of high-dependency areas for selected patients is not associated with increased morbidity and mortality.

Major vascular surgery is associated with significant third space fluid losses and central venous pressure monitoring is essential postoperatively. The use of pulmonary artery catheters to optimize volume replacement has no effect on morbidity or mortality. An adequate circulating volume must be maintained to protect vital organs, particularly the kidneys and gut. Inotropic therapy may be required initially if acidosis and hypothermia are causing myocardial depression. Ventilation may be required for the first few hours.

Coagulopathy is common and a clotting profile should be sent routinely and abnormalities treated appropriately. Many patients with vascular disease take aspirin or clopidogrel which cause platelet dysfunction. Haematocrit should be maintained around 30% with appropriate combinations of blood, colloid and crystalloid. Thrombosis and graft occlusion are serious complications and prophylaxis is important. Low-molecular-weight heparin is routinely prescribed and heparin given during surgery is often not reversed to maintain some degree of anticoagulation in the early postoperative period.

Many patients are hypothermic and need to be gradually rewarmed using a forced-air warming device. As the patient rewarms, vasoconstriction is replaced by vasodilation and hypotension may occur. Enteral feeding should be commenced as early as day two. Multi-organ failure is more common after emergency aneurysm surgery. Contributory factors include prolonged periods of hypotension or cardiac arrest during surgery, hypoperfusion resulting in acidosis and massive transfusion.

Epidural analgesia provides excellent pain relief during the postoperative period and a combination of local anaesthetics and opioids can be infused for several days, if necessary. Vasodilation requires careful management with fluids and vasconstrictors. Motor block may hinder mobilization and regular neurological observations should be performed. If regional techniques are inappropriate, then patient-controlled analgesia with morphine is used, supplemented with paracetamol and non-steroidal anti-inflammatory drugs, providing there are no contraindications to the latter.

Perioperative myocardial infarction is the commonest cause of death after vascular surgery with an incidence of 2% to 5%. Myocardial infarction should be suspected in any patient with cardiovascular instability that does not respond to simple interventions, and is diagnosed by serial 12-lead ECG and measurement of cardiac enzymes. Treatment should follow standard practice but thrombolysis is contraindicated in the early postoperative period. There are a number of possible causes for myocardial ischaemia, including increased myocardial oxygen demand in the presence of impaired coronary blood flow, hypercoagulability of blood and nocturnal hypoxaemia.

Carotid endarterectomy

Atherosclerosis is the commonest cause of carotid artery occlusive disease. Risk factors for development of the disease include male gender, age > 70 years, hypertension and smoking. The prevalence of significant carotid artery stenosis is higher in patients with left mainstem coronary artery disease and those with peripheral vascular disease. Surgery is indicated for patients with > 70% stenosis and significant symptoms. Patients at highest risk from surgery are those with unstable neurological symptoms and extensive medical comorbidity. Perioperative mortality from myocardial infarction or stroke is approximately 5%.

The two main goals of anaesthesia during carotid endarterectomy (CEA) are to protect the brain and the heart but these goals may conflict. Either general or regional anaesthesia can be used, and each has its advocates. A comparison of general and regional anaesthesia for carotid endarterectomy is shown in Table 8.9. At present, there is no good evidence to favour one technique over the other.

General anaesthesia

The aims are to maintain haemodynamic stability and cerebral perfusion whilst reducing cerebral oxygen consumption. Normal blood pressure should be maintained with the judicious use of vasopressors where

Table 8.9 Comparison of local and general anaesthesia for carotid endarterectomy

General anaesthesia	Local anaesthesia
Reduces cerebral oxygen consumption	Excellent analgesia
Isoflurane improves cerebral blood flow	Patient acts as own monitor
Control of $PaCO_2$	Reduced respiratory complications
Good patient tolerance	Block complications
Quiet surgical field for surgeon	Patient may refuse
Good control of the airway	
Hypertension at extubation	

necessary. Controlled ventilation ensures the partial pressure of carbon dioxide in blood remains within normal limits. The choice of drug to induce and maintain anaesthesia has not been shown to affect outcome.

Active cooling is not used but the temperature often falls to around 35°C which may provide some cerebral protection. It is essential for the patient to awaken quickly at the end of the procedure so that neurological assessment can be undertaken. Tracheal intubation and extubation may cause significant hypertension which can result in a sudden undesirable rise in cerebral perfusion pressure. Strategies aimed at avoiding this include intravenous antihypertensives such as esmolol or labetalol, opioids, and deep extubation followed by mask ventilation or insertion of a Laryngeal Mask Airway™ whilst the patient is still paralysed.

In addition to standard non-invasive monitoring, invasive arterial pressure monitoring is routine for CEA. Attention has been paid towards cerebral function monitoring during carotid endarterectomy to assess the adequacy of the collateral circulation during cross-clamping (Table 8.10). An awake patient precludes the need for cerebral monitoring because changes in speech or mentation during cross-clamping indicate that a shunt is required.

Local anaesthesia

Regional anaesthesia is widely used for CEA. Sensory blockade in the C2–C4 dermatome can be achieved in several ways, by superficial or deep cervical plexus block or subcutaneous infiltration of the peripheral nerves. These nerves have a common point of emergence around the mid-point of the sternocleidomastoid muscle and are relatively accessible. Blocks used include:

• Superficial cervical plexus block: a simple technique with unilateral effects.
• Deep cervical plexus block: more difficult to perform than superficial block, but provides better analgesia. Both intravascular and

---

Table 8.10   Methods of monitoring cerebral function during carotid endarterectomy

Electroencephalography
Somatosensory evoked potentials
Transcranial Doppler ultrasound
Carotid artery stump pressure measurement

subarachnoid injections can occur. Side-effects include haematoma, hoarseness, stellate ganglion block, phrenic nerve block and Horner's syndrome.

- Cervical epidural: all cervical and upper thoracic nerve roots are blocked which may cause hypotension, bradycardia and respiratory failure.

Problems may occur if regional blockade is not complete, the incision extends into an area supplied by the cranial nerves, or pain arises from the carotid sheath. Local anaesthetic supplementation may be undertaken or sedation administered with a low-dose propofol infusion ensuring that the patient is able to cooperate and communicate.

Postoperative care (Table 8.11)

Many patients can be transferred back to the ward after a period of observation in a recovery area provided that appropriate observations are made regularly. Most patients requiring interventions, or with adverse outcomes, can be identified within the first 8 h postoperatively. High-risk patients, such as those with previous stroke or myocardial infarction, should be monitored in an HDU initially.

Both hypertension and hypotension are common in the early postoperative period. The cause of postoperative hypertension is unclear, but may result from malfunction of baroreceptors in the carotid sinus nerve, and is associated with more neurological deficits. Blood pressure should be maintained at preoperative levels. Hypotension may also occur, probably due to increased firing of the carotid sinus nerve, together with a vagally mediated bradycardia. It usually resolves within 12–24 h but should be treated with fluids and vasopressors to maintain diastolic coronary perfusion pressure. Local anaesthetic instilled at surgery may prevent this complication.

Table 8.11   Complications following carotid endarterectomy

Haemodynamic instability
Onset of new neurological dysfunction: focal deficits
Hyperperfusion syndrome
Wound haematoma
Cranial nerve damage
Respiratory insufficiency

Patients emerging from surgery with a new neurological deficit require immediate surgical review. Postoperative neurological observation should be carried out every 15 min and any change in condition should be regarded as an indication for Doppler ultrasound examination of the carotid artery. Sixty to seventy percent of strokes occur perioperatively and usually result from embolic episodes. More than 10% of patients suffer various cranial nerve injuries from surgical manipulation, including the recurrent laryngeal nerve, the hypoglossal nerve and the facial nerve.

Hyperperfusion syndrome results from blood flow to the brain in excess of its metabolic needs. The syndrome does not occur for several days after surgery and presents with ipsilateral headache, unresponsive to treatment, and may progress to cerebral excitability and fits. The cause is unknown.

Postoperative respiratory insufficiency may be caused by bilateral recurrent laryngeal nerve palsy, massive haematoma or abnormal carotid body function. A rapidly expanding haematoma may compromise the airway due to venous and lymphatic obstruction resulting in pharyngeal oedema and should be evacuated urgently. Postoperative bleeding is more common if a vein patch is used.

Postoperative analgesia is not a major problem. In patients with a cervical plexus block, no further analgesia will be required. However, patients awakening from general anaesthesia may initially require morphine.

Percutaneous endovascular procedures

Percutaneous revascularization for peripheral vascular disease was first described in 1964. Currently, percutanous transluminal angioplasty (PTA) uses a variety of devices, ranging from implantable stents to endovascular radiation devices for restenosis. Peripheral angioplasty can be performed with local anaesthesia in high-risk patients with low morbidity and mortality. Recovery is rapid and patients can return to normal activity soon after the procedure. Endovascular stent techniques have been applied to both abdominal and thoracic aortic aneurysms with good results in selected patients. A reduced need for blood products, and a lower incidence of respiratory and renal failure compared with patients undergoing open surgery, has been demonstrated, but there is no difference in cardiac complications or mortality. Anaesthetic techniques include general anaesthesia, regional anaesthesia and direct local infiltration of the access site in the femoral artery.

PTA and stenting can also be used to treat carotid stenosis under local anaesthesia. Complications include intimal dissection and plaque rupture. Trial data showed no difference in the incidence of disabling stroke or death within 30 days of treatment between patients randomized to surgery or endovascular treatment. Complications such as cranial nerve palsy and haematoma were less common in the endovascular group, but restenosis was more common.

The anaesthetist is most likely to be involved with the insertion of abdominal or thoracic endovascular stents. Endovascular aortic aneurysm repair involves transfemoral placement of an intraluminal prosthetic graft into the aorta with the aim of excluding the aneurysm sac from the circulation. This is usually undertaken in a radiology suite with surgeons available. There are implications for anaesthesia in terms of availability of equipment, assistance, monitoring and temperature control. General or regional anaesthesia can be used, but the administration of heparin and the potential for a prolonged procedure cause many anaesthetists to favour general anaesthesia. Full monitoring and adequate vascular access are essential. Blood loss from the femoral arteriotomy site can be significant and all patients should be cross-matched. The aorta is only occluded for a short period while the stent is opened. Haemodynamic instability is not a problem in patients undergoing endovascular repair. Normotension is maintained throughout the procedure, except during balloon inflation when a reduction in arterial pressure is required to prevent the stent moving. Many patients have impaired renal function, and the use of large volumes of contrast media means that urine output should be carefully monitored. Most patients can be woken at the end of the procedure and transferred to an HDU.

Further reading

Bender JS, Smith-Meek MA, Jones CE. Routine pulmonary artery catheterisation does not reduce morbidity and mortality of elective vascular surgery: results of a prospective randomised trial. Ann Surg 1997;226:229–236.

Bew S, Bryant A, Desborough J, Hall G. Epidural analgesia and arterial reconstructive surgery to the leg: effects on fibrinolysis and platelet degranulation. Br J Anaesth 2000;86:230–235.

Bayly PJ, Matthews JN, Dobson PM, Price ML, Thomas DG. In-hospital mortality from abdominal aortic surgery in Great Britain and Ireland: Vascular Anaesthesia Society Audit. Br J Surg 2001;88:687–692.

Bode R, Lewis K, Zarich S, Pierce ET, Roberts M, Kowalchuk GJ, Satwicz PR, Gibbons GW, Hunter JA, Espanola CC. Cardiac outcome after peripheral vascular surgery: comparison of general and regional anaesthesia. Anesthesiology 1996;84:3–13.

Caldicott L, Lumb A, McCoy D. Vascular anaesthesia: a practical hand book. Oxford: Butterworth Heinemann; 2000.

Dutch Bypass Oral Anticoagulants or Aspirin (BOA) Study group. Efficacy of oral anticoagulation compared with aspirin after infra-inguinal bypass surgery: a randomised trial. Lancet 2000;355:346–351.

Grieff JM, Thompson M, Langham. Anaesthetic implications of aortic stent surgery. Br J Anaesth 1995;75:779–781.

Nott DM, Crinnion J, Benson J, Came A, Gunning P. Laparoscopically assisted abdominal aortic aneurysm repair. Lancet 1999;353:1765–1766.

Riambau V, Laheij RJ, Garcia-Madrid C, Sanchez-Espin; EUROSTAR group. The association between co-morbidity and mortality after abdominal aortic aneurysm endografting in patients ineligible for elective open surgery. Eur J Endovasc Surg 2001;22:265–270.

Tangkanakul C, Counsell C, Warlow C. Local versus general anaesthesia for carotid endarterectomy. Cochrane Database System Rev 2000;2:CD000126.

9

Preoperative assessment of the thoracic surgical patient

The majority of lung resections are carried out for the treatment of primary malignant lung tumours (Table 9.1). Mortality for pulmonary resection remains relatively high at 5% for pneumonectomy and 2.9% for lobectomy. Lung resection inevitably leads to loss of functioning lung tissue except on the rare occasion when the disease has already destroyed the lobe, or lung, to be removed. The assessment of pre-operative lung function is of great importance in these patients. This chapter concentrates on the assessment of patients undergoing lung resection but an increasing number of patients (Table 9.1) undergo video-assisted thoracoscopic surgery. It is notable that patients pre-senting for other forms of thoracic surgery may have greater impair-ment of lung function. Those undergoing lung volume reduction surgery, lung biopsy and lung transplantation may all have very poor lung function.

General anaesthetic assessment

The patient presenting for lung resection will have been fully evaluated by the appropriate medical and surgical teams before surgery. The anaesthetist should briefly review their findings and, where necessary, investigate factors specifically relevant to anaesthesia (see Chapter 1). It is important to continue bronchodilator therapy up to and including the morning of operation. Many of these patients will also have pre-existing cardiovascular disease and therefore anti-anginal therapy and antihypertensive medication should be continued. Aspirin and non-steroidal anti-inflammatory drugs are discontinued at least 1 week before surgery.

The anaesthetist should note any features which suggest difficult tracheal intubation because these problems are often compounded when bulky and cumbersome endobronchial tubes have to be inserted. The site and position of the trachea should be ascertained clinically and on chest X-ray, and any distortion of the main bronchi also noted as these

Table 9.1 Thoracic surgical results from 47 UK centres (1999–2000). (Adapted from the database of the Society of Cardiothoracic Surgeons of Great Britain and Ireland.)

Operation	Numbers	Deaths	Mortality (%)
Lung resection: primary malignant tumours			
Pneumonectomy	779	39	5.0
Lobectomy/bilobectomy	2208	63	2.9
Video-assisted thoracoscopic surgery: pulmonary/pleural disease			
Lung biopsy	506	6	1.2
Bullae	56	2	3.6
Lung volume reduction surgery			
Unilateral	50	3	6.0
Bilateral	15	1	6.7
Pneumothorax (various procedures)	735	6	0.8
Pleural biopsy	499	5	1.0
Pleural biopsy + chemical pleurodesis	932	18	1.9
Pleurectomy	84	2	2.4
Pleurectomy + drainage empyema	154	4	2.6

may affect endobronchial intubation. It is also useful to look for physical features such as a short neck and abnormal body-build which may influence the choice and size of endobronchial tube. Abnormalities of the cervical, thoracic and lumbar spine may make positioning of the patient in the lateral thoracotomy position difficult or dangerous. Hyperextension of the neck in the supine position for bronchoscopy or mediastinoscopy is particularly hazardous in the presence of an unstable cervical spine.

An intercostal drain may be present in certain circumstances, when the quantity of blood, pus or air draining should be noted.

General investigations
All patients require, as a minimum, a recent chest X-ray, an electrocardiogram, full blood count and urea and electrolyte measurements, liver function tests and preoperative blood cross-match. Baseline lung function tests are essential in all patients but some patients may need more extensive tests of cardiorespiratory function.

Assessment of the cardiovascular system
Many patients, presenting for lung resection will be relatively elderly and lifelong smokers. Not suprisingly, morbidity and mortality from cardiovascular disease is common after thoracic surgery. The Goldman Multifactorial Risk Index has been used to quantify the cardiovascular risk associated with non-cardiac surgery (see Chapter 7) More recently, the American College of Cardiology and the American Heart Association have published guidelines for perioperative cardiovascular evaluation for non-cardiac surgery (see Chapter 7). Clinical predictors of increased perioperative cardiovascular risk estimated in this review are detailed in Table 9.2. Intrathoracic surgery is considered to be an intermediate risk for cardiac death and non-fatal myocardial infarction.

Cardiac dysfunction is particularly relevant following pneumonectomy where the whole of the cardiac output has to pass through one remaining lung. Significant pulmonary hypertension and right heart failure due to lung disease are likely to preclude major lung resection, but lesser degrees of pulmonary vascular disease may be tolerated. Direct measurement of pulmonary artery pressure is rarely undertaken preoperatively as cardiorespiratory function can be investigated more easily, although less specifically, by exercise testing and to some extent by the measurement of maximum breathing capacity.

Table 9.2   Clinical predictors of increased perioperative cardiovascular risk. (Adapted from the American College of Cardiology/American Heart Association guidelines for perioperative evaluation for non-cardiac surgery 1996.)

Major

Unstable coronary syndromes
  Recent myocardial infarction with evidence of important ischaemic risk by clinical symptoms or non-invasive study
  Unstable or severe angina (Canadian class III or IV)
Decompensated congestive heart failure
Significant arrhythmias
  High-grade atrioventricular block
  Symptomatic ventricular arrhythmias in the presence of underlying heart disease
  Supraventricular arrhythmias with uncontrolled ventricular rate
Severe valvular disease

Intermediate

Mild angina pectoris (Canadian class I or II)
Prior myocardial infarction by history or pathological Q waves
Compensated or prior congestive heart failure
Diabetes mellitus

Minor

Advanced age
Abnormal electrocardiogram (left ventricular hypertrophy, left bundle branch block)
ST abnormalities
Rhythm other than sinus (e.g. atrial fibrillation)
Low functional capacity (e.g. inability to climb one flight of stairs)
History of stroke
Uncontrolled systemic hypertension

Assessment of the respiratory system
Clinical history
The clinical history is of great importance in the initial diagnosis of chest diseases. Symptoms of dyspnoea and haemoptysis are relevant to anaesthesia.

Dyspnoea is subjective and difficult to quantify by direct questioning. An active patient with no significant exercise limitation is likely to tolerate lung resection and even pneumonectomy. A patient whose exercise capacity is severely limited (e.g. only able to climb one flight of stairs without stopping) may not tolerate lung resection and requires careful evaluation. Patients who are breathless at rest are unlikely to tolerate lung resection. Minor haemoptysis is not usually worrying in the cancer patient but may predict intraoperative bleeding. Major haemoptysis is uncommon with operable malignant lesions but can, very rarely, necessitate emergency lung resection. Haemoptysis due to cavitating tuberculosis, aspergilloma and arteriovenous malformations is much more worrying and potentially difficult to deal with surgically.

Physical examination
The physical examination is aimed at the points of anaesthetic interest discussed above. In addition, auscultation of the chest may reveal further information, such as the presence of wheeze, which will aid interpretation of the preoperative chest X-ray and lung function tests.

Chest X-ray
Inspection of a postero–anterior and lateral chest X-ray will show the site of any localized lesion and its relationship to the hilum, mediastinum and chest wall. These X-rays, together with the computerized tomography (CT) scan, should be in the anaesthetic room before induction of anaesthesia.

The direction, shape and diameter of the trachea and main bronchi may alert the anaesthetist to potential problems with endobronchial intubation. Almost invariably, more than one imaging technique is required to assess the extent and operability of lung cancer.

Computerized tomography
CT scanning, and the faster scanning techniques, are now an established method of demonstrating lesions within the thorax, some of which cannot be readily demonstrated by conventional radiology. CT scanning, with contrast enhancement, is used to identify the site, size and possible extension of intrathoracic tumours originating in the

lungs and hilum. Patients with primary lung cancer are accepted for surgery, provided there are no distant metastases and there is no evidence of nodal spread. Those with hilar and mediastinal lymphadenopathy undergo mediastinoscopy and biopsy of these nodes. If the nodes are invaded with tumour, the patient is unlikely to be curable by lung resection.

CT scanning may include the brain, liver and adrenals to search for metastatic disease.

Magnetic resonance imaging
Magnetic resonance imaging techniques have not proved superior to CT scanning for the investigation of intrathoracic pathology.

Positron emission tomography
2-[f-18]fluoro-2-deoxy-D-glucose (FDG) has an increased uptake in malignant cells. Positron emission tomography using FDG is a non-invasive imaging technique which has been found to be highly accurate in differentiating benign from malignant solitary pulmonary nodules and lung lesions.

Other scanning techniques
Bone scan
Radioisotope scanning techniques are used in patients with lung cancer who have bone pain or significant weight loss to detect bony secondaries.

Liver scan
A CT scan may show liver abnormalities but, if this is not diagnostic, a liver ultrasound can differentiate between cystic and solid lesions.

Lung function tests
Arterial gas analysis
We routinely measure arterial gas values with the patient breathing room air preoperatively, as a baseline. Arterial hypoxaemia is a poor indicator of risk of lung resection. In thoracic surgery, the portion of lung to be removed may be contributing to a physiological shunt with persistent blood flow but little or no ventilation, although this is offset to some extent by the compensatory mechanism of hypoxic pulmonary vasoconstriction. In marginal cases, this can be investigated by ventilation–perfusion scanning techniques. It is also important to remember that arterial oxygen tension declines with age, the lower limit for

normal in the 70–79 year-old age group is 9 kPa and just above 10 kPa for the 50–59 year-old age group.

A $PaCO_2 > 6$ kPa represents increased perioperative risk of pulmonary complications and mortality. This level of hypercapnia is not an absolute contraindication to lung resection.

Bedside spirometry

Relatively fit patients with good exercise tolerance only need baseline measurements of forced vital capacity (FVC) and forced expiratory volume in 1 s (FEV_1). These can be carried out at the bedside or in the outpatient clinic. If the FEV_1 is > 2 l and the FVC > 50% of predicted values, the patient is likely to tolerate pneumonectomy and no further lung function testing will be required. If values fall significantly below these figures, particularly if FEV_1 approaches 1 l, it is necessary to carry out formal lung function testing in the laboratory.

Laboratory lung function testing

Formal pulmonary function testing allows accurate measurement of static and dynamic lung volumes and other indices of lung function, such as gas transfer. These measurements are carried out before, and after, bronchodilator therapy and the results compared with normal values related to age, sex, size and ethnic origin. A variety of indices indicate increased risk after lung resection (Table 9.3) but the main criterion is the FEV_1. A FEV_1 of 800–1000 ml is required to produce an effective cough to aid clearance of secretions. In a patient of average size, a FEV_1 of 1 l is associated with a reasonable chance of surviving pneumonectomy without a significant risk of respiratory failure postoperatively. Some surgeons consider that a 'predicted' postoperative FEV_1 of 800–1000 ml is the limit for pneumonectomy. This is calculated on the basis of functional losses (in relation to preoperative

Table 9.3   Summary of criteria considered to indicate increased risk of morbidity or mortality following lung resection

Forced vital capacity	< 50% predicted
Forced expiratory volume in 1 s	< 2.0 l or 50% predicted
Maximum breathing capacity	< 50% predicted
$PaCO_2$	> 6.0 kPa
Residual volume/total lung capacity ratio	< 50% predicted
Carbon monoxide gas transfer	< 50% predicted

values) of 25% for lobectomy or 33% for pneumonectomy. More accurate predictions can be made using preoperative radioisotope ventilation–perfusion scanning techniques.

In patients with a marginal FEV_1, the measurement of maximum breathing capacity (MBC) or formal exercise testing provides additional information.

Maximum breathing capacity
MBC is obtained by a period of voluntary hyperventilation through a low resistance circuit for 15 s. Motivation, sustainable muscle strength and low airway resistance contribute to successful performance of this test. As these factors are important in postoperatively, it is not surprising that the test is predictive of morbidity and mortality. Patients with an MBC < 50% of the predicted value are at increased risk of hospital mortality.

Exercise testing
When patients have a peak oxygen uptake, during exercise < 15 ml/kg/min, the risk of postoperative complications increases.

However, some studies have found no predictive value of exercise testing in lung resection.

Assessment of the lung resection patient
The assessment of the lung resection patient focuses on the cardio-vascular and respiratory systems. Minimum levels of lung function for various operations are summarized in Table 9.4. and a practical approach to preoperative assessment is summarized in Fig. 9.1. In general, no patient should be denied surgery on the basis of a single lung function test.

The final decision about surgery is usually made by the surgeon after routine laboratory pulmonary function testing.

Preoperative preparation
Fit patients need little preoperative preparation but they should be instructed by a physiotherapist in the breathing exercises and coughing which will be required postoperatively.

Smokers should be encouraged to stop preoperatively. Cessation of smoking is followed by a decrease in the volume of mucus hypersecretion and airway reactivity, as well as improved mucociliary transport. These beneficial effects may lessen the incidence of postoperative atelectasis and infection but take 2–4 weeks to develop. The short term

Table 9.4   Suggested whole lung pulmonary function criteria for lung resection. (Adapted from Thomas et al. 1995.)

Test	Pneumonectomy	Lobectomy	Wedge/segment
Maximum breathing capacity (% predicted)	> 55	> 40	> 35
Forced expiratory volume in 1 s (l)	> 2*	> 1	> 0.6
Forced expiratory volume in 1 s (% predicted)	> 55	40–50	> 35–40

* Accepting this value as absolute lower limit for pneumonectomy may be unduly pessimistic (see Fig. 9.1)

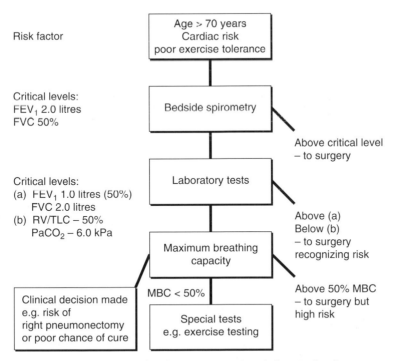

Figure 9.1   Risk factors and pulmonary resection. (After Gothard J, Kelleher A. Essentials of cardiac and thoracic anaesthesia. Oxford: Butterworth Heinemann; 1999, with permission.)

effects of stopping smoking (48–72 h) may be associated with increased secretions and hyperactive airways. However, there will be a decrease in carboxyhaemoglobin content of the blood and better oxygen delivery to the tissues.

More attention should be given to the preparation of patients with poor lung function, particularly if there is a treatable component to their disease, such as reversible airway obstruction, infected sputum or a source of reinfection in the sinuses or teeth.

Drugs which can be used to relieve bronchospasm include sympathomimetic agents, oral theophylline derivatives, ipratropium bromide (atrovent) and inhaled corticosteroids, such as beclomethasone dipropionate. In patients not already on bronchodilator therapy, we use salbutamol with ipratropium by nebulizer preoperatively.

Patients with lung cancer and a chest infection may require antibiotic treatment before admission to hospital. Those with a chronic pulmonary infection may require admission to hospital for several days preoperatively so that sputum can be cultured, appropriate antibiotics given and physiotherapy started.

Premedication

After a sympathetic explanation of perioperative events, and a discussion of analgesic techniques to be used postoperatively, most patients are calm and satisfactorily sedated after temazepam (10–20 mg) orally 1–2 h before surgery. Oral hydration, with clear fluids only up to 2 h preoperatively, is encouraged. If hypersecretion becomes a problem, glycopyrronium is given intravenously during surgery.

Ancillary drug therapy

All relevant medication is continued up to the time of surgery.

Most patients are given low-molecular-weight heparin subcutaneously, starting on the morning of operation and continuing into the postoperative period.

Antibiotic prophylaxis is started immediately after the induction of anaesthesia and continued for 24 h.

Further reading

American College of Cardiology/American Heart Association guidelines for perioperative evaluation for noncardiac surgery. Circulation 1996;93: 1278–1317.

Crapo RO. Pulmonary-function testing. Current concepts. N Engl J Med 1994;331:25–30.

Goldman L. Cardiac risk in noncardiac surgery: an update. Anesth Analg 1995; 80:810–820.

Mangano DT. Perioperative cardiac morbidity. Anesthesiology 1990;72: 153–184.

Slinger PD, Johnston MR. Preoperative assessment for pulmonary resection. J Cardiothorac Vasc Anesth 2000;14:202–211.

Smetana GW. Preoperative pulmonary evaluation. Current concepts. N Engl J Med 1999;340:937–944.

Thomas SD, Berry PD, Russell GN. Is this patient fit for thoracotomy and resection of lung tissue? Postgrad Med J 1995;71:331–335.

10

Anaesthesia for thoracic surgery

Anaesthetic techniques

Anaesthetic techniques for thoracic surgery (Table 10.1) are little different from those used in other forms of major surgery. Anaesthesia is induced intravenously and endobronchial intubation is performed following the administration of a non-depolarizing neuromuscular blocking drug. The depolarizing agent suxamethonium is indicated, however, if a difficult laryngeal intubation is likely, or if another airway problem, such as a bronchopleural fistula, is present.

Maintenance of anaesthesia is usually with an inhalational agent such as isoflurane, combined with an intravenous opioid, but it is equally acceptable to use a total intravenous technique.

If epidural opioids are to be used to provide postoperative pain relief, then it is preferable to avoid the use of intravenous opioids during surgery. Postoperative analgesia is discussed in Chapter 12.

The choice between inhalational anaesthesia and intravenous techniques during one-lung ventilation is controversial. In practice, there is little difference in the oxygenation achieved with each technique.

Monitoring

Monitoring and vascular access for major thoracic surgery should be comprehensive, (Table 10.2). A pulmonary artery catheter is unnecessary in routine practice.

Isolation of the lungs

Separation of the lungs to facilitate one-lung ventilation (OLV) and prevent spread of secretions, pus and blood from one lung to other is usually achieved with a double-lumen endobronchial tube (DLT). The advent of video-assisted thoracoscopic surgery (VATS) has increased the use of endobronchial intubation because it is mandatory to collapse the lung on the side of thoracoscopic surgery to allow safe access via telescope and instrumentation ports. There has also been a resurgence of interest in the use of bronchial blockade, particularly with the Univent tube.

Table 10.1   Anaesthetic techniques suitable for major thoracic surgery

Induction
Propofol
Satisfactory in most patients; repeat, as necessary, to prevent awareness during preoperative bronchoscopy.
Target-controlled infusion useful for longer procedures and prolonged bronchoscopy
Etomidate
Elderly or those with cardiovascular instability

Neuromuscular blockade
Choice of non-depolarizing agent not critical
Consider suxamethonium for difficult intubation, or airway fistula

Maintenance of anaesthesia
Inhalational agent
Isoflurance most suitable
Avoid halothane: has marked inhibitory effect on hypoxic pulmonary vasoconstriction
Inspired gas mixture: 50% oxygen in nitrous oxide or air
Avoid nitrous oxide with abnormal air spaces
Increase inspired oxygen concentration for one-lung ventilat on (air/oxygen combination preferable)
Total intravenous anaesthesia
Propofol by target controlled infusion: combine with remifentanil infusion?
Intraoperative analgesia
Morphine (0.1–0.2 mg/kg) based on age/physical status, etc., supplement at end of surgery
Fentanyl (5–15 μg/kg): alternative
Avoid intravenous opioids if epidural opioids used
Epidural analgesia
Thoracic/high lumbar/lumbar: all feasible
Opioids alone or combined with low-dose local anaesthetic agents

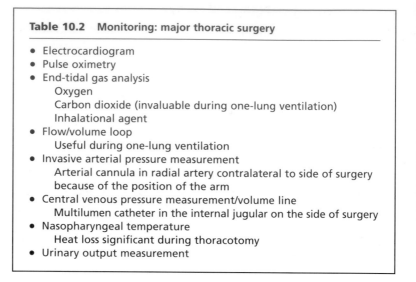

Table 10.2   Monitoring: major thoracic surgery

- Electrocardiogram
- Pulse oximetry
- End-tidal gas analysis
  - Oxygen
  - Carbon dioxide (invaluable during one-lung ventilation)
  - Inhalational agent
- Flow/volume loop
  - Useful during one-lung ventilation
- Invasive arterial pressure measurement
  - Arterial cannula in radial artery contralateral to side of surgery because of the position of the arm
- Central venous pressure measurement/volume line
  - Multilumen catheter in the internal jugular on the side of surgery
- Nasopharyngeal temperature
  - Heat loss significant during thoracotomy
- Urinary output measurement

Endobronchial intubation

It is preferable to use a left-sided DLT whenever possible because this avoids the problem of the early 'take-off' of the right upper lobe bronchus. A left-sided DLT can be used for the majority of VATS procedures, but it is accepted UK practice to place a DLT in the lung contralateral to surgery to facilitate lung resection. Indications for endobronchial intubation theoretically range from absolute to relative (Table 10.3).

Table 10.3   Indications for endobronchial intubation

Absolute	Fistula or ruptured airway
	Lung transplantation
	Video-assisted thoracoscopic surgery
	Intrapulmonary bleeding
	Profuse secretions
	Lung cysts
	Lung resection
	Thoracic aortic/spinal surgery
	Oesophageal surgery
Relative	Open pleurectomy

In practice, one-lung ventilation is used to facilitate all the above procedures if satisfactory oxygenation can be maintained.

Double-lumen endobronchial tubes

DLTs are derived from the Carlens tube which was introduced in 1949 to allow measurement of lung volumes separately in the two lungs (differential bronchospirometry).

The majority of tubes available are based on a design by the British anaesthetist Robertshaw and incorporate an endobronchial limb, a tracheal limb and both tracheal and bronchial cuffs. They are shaped to fit into the airway with a proximal oropharyngeal curve and a distal bronchial curve. The bronchial cuff design is different between the left and right tubes because the right upper lobe orifice occurs a shorter distance after the carina than the left upper lobe orifice (Fig. 10.1). Most right tubes have a ventilation slot (or similar arrangement) built into, or distal to, the right bronchial cuff for right upper lobe ventilation. Left tubes do not have this feature because of the longer left main bronchus. The basic pattern of a right DLT is shown in Fig 10.2. Endobronchial tubes are made to a similar pattern by numerous different manufacturers.

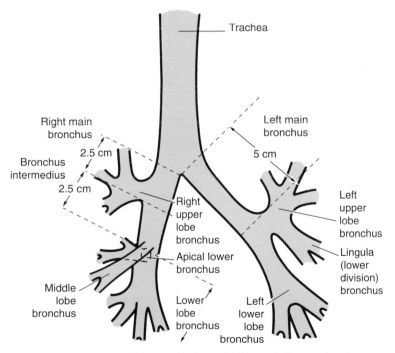

Figure 10.1 Anatomy of the tracheobronchial tree. (After Gothard J, Kelleher A. Essentials of Cardiac and thoracic anaesthesia. Oxford: Butterworth Heinemann; 1999, with permission.)

Table 10.4 lists the features of two types of endobronchial tube (Robertshaw and Bronchocath) commonly used in the UK.

The size of tube to be used, and depth of insertion of certain tubes, is based to some extent on the age, weight, height and sex of the patient

Table 10.4 Comparison of Robertshaw and Bronchocath endobronchial tubes

Robertshaw (Phoenix Medical Ltd)	Bronchocath (Mallinckrodt)
Construction Disposable (coated rubber) also red rubber reusable Bronchial limb and cuff colour-coded blue	**Construction** Polyvinylchloride Disposable Low-pressure/high volume cuffs Colour-coded blue bronchial cuff and bronchial limb Radio-opaque markings
Sizes Right and left Large, medium, small, extra-small	**Sizes** Right and left 35, 37, 39 and 41-French gauge Left 28-French gauge
Features 'Bite-block' where tracheal and bronchial limbs fuse is designed to sit at level of teeth; in practice this may be too deep Slot in bronchial cuff (21 mm – large tube) almost twice the length of equivalent Bronchocath, therefore more likely to be opposite the right upper lobe orifice	**Features** Depth of insertion variable Length markers on side of tube Right upper lobe ventilation slot only 11 mm in 41-French gauge tube Easier to use with fibreoptic bronchoscope. Standard anaesthetic fibreoptic bronchoscope will pass down 35-French gauge tube
Clinical use Relatively bulky tubes, easy to insert and less likely to move intraoperatively than plastic tubes Less easy to manipulate with a fibreoptic bronchoscope. The small and extra-small sizes will only allow passage of a paediatric fibreoptic bronchoscope	**Clinical use** Not as stable after insertion as Robertshaw tube Greater size range useful, especially in small women/ adolescents Malleable plastic tubes useful for 'rail-roading' techniques with a fibreoptic bronchoscope and difficult laryngeal intubation

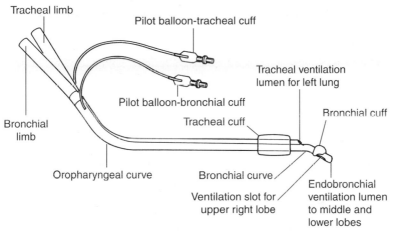

Figure 10.2   Basic pattern of a right-sided double-lumen endobronchial tube. (After Gothard J. Anaesthesia for thoracic surgery, 2nd edn. Oxford: Blackwell Scientific Publications; 1993, with permission.)

(Table 10.5). Once the initial choice of tube is in place, its position is checked clinically and by fibreoptic bronchoscopy (FOB) and this may indicate that a different size of tube is necessary.

Placement of double-lumen endobronchial tubes

DLTs are usually placed in the lung contralateral to surgery but, as discussed above, left-sided tubes are placed where possible for

Table 10.5   Recommendations for size and length of left double-lumen tube. (Adapted from Brodsky et al. 1991, 1996.)

Length of tube
Male/females 170 cm tall: insert tube to a depth of 29 cm
For every 10 cm increase in height, increase depth of insertion by 1 cm

Size of tube from measured tracheal width

Width of trachea (mm)	Tube size (French gauge)
18	41
16	39
15	37
14	35

The above lengths and sizes are not necessarily applicable to right-sided tubes.

other types of surgery to overcome the problem of right upper lobe ventilation.

DLTs are introduced into the larynx in the usual way, sometimes aided with a bougie. The tube is then advanced 'blindly' (after removing any stilette provided) with a twisting motion towards the side of insertion. The curved endobronchial portion of the tube is usually deflected at the carina and passes into the appropriate main bronchus.

Once in place, the tracheal cuff is inflated whilst both lungs are ventilated and the seal checked in the usual way. The tracheal limb of the DLT is then opened to air and the double-lumen catheter mount clamped so that only the bronchial limb is ventilated. The bronchial cuff is then inflated with a minimum amount of air to seal the cuff and eliminate any leak of gas from the intubated lung up through the open tracheal limb. This step is important for two reasons. First, a good seal is required to establish satisfactory one-lung anaesthesia during surgery and, second, bronchial rupture has been reported after overinflation of the bronchial cuff.

During this process, the position of the tube is checked by observing chest movements with inflation/deflation and by alternate auscultation of both lung fields, paying particular attention to the left upper lobe with a left-sided tube and the right upper lobe with a right-sided tube. Auscultation is also carried out first with the tracheal limb, and then the endobronchial limb, occluded at the catheter mount to ascertain that isolation of the lungs has been achieved. Finally, the change in airway pressure is noted when OLV is started. These checks are repeated after the patient has been turned into the lateral position for thoracotomy, because it is not uncommon for the tube to move at this time.

There is increasing evidence that clinical checks of tube position are inaccurate and that it is preferable to check the position of endobronchial tubes with an FOB.

Fibreoptic bronchoscopy and double-lumen tube placement

The introduction of slim, relatively inexpensive, FOB/laryngoscopes has made the routine inspection of endobronchial tubes a practical possibility.

The FOB can be used to place the endobronchial tube under direct vision in patients who are difficult to intubate, or when the tube cannot be located blindly in the appropriate bronchus. In the latter situation, it is a relatively simple task to insert a DLT into the trachea, locate the appropriate main bronchus with an FOB passed down the tube and then 'railroad' or slide the tube into position over the bronchoscope

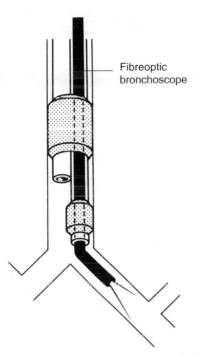

Fibreoptic
bronchoscope

Figure 10.3 Positioning of a double-lumen tube with the fibre-optic bronchoscope. (After Aitkenhead AR, Jones RM. Clinical anaesthesia. Edinburgh: Churchill Livingstone; 1996, with permission.)

(Fig. 10.3). The flexibility of plastic tubes is a distinct advantage when the FOB is used in this way.

In the majority of cases, the FOB will be used to check the position of tubes following blind placement. The sequence for checking the position of a DLT is described below.

The FOB (Fig 10.4) is first passed down the tracheal lumen of the DLT to check that there is a clear view of the main bronchus of the lung to be operated upon and that the bronchial cuff is not herniating over the carina. (The bronchial cuff of the majority of tubes is coloured blue for easy endoscopic identification.) The FOB is then passed down the endobronchial limb to ensure that the upper lobe orifice is not obstructed on the left and that the ventilation slot of a right tube is apposed to the upper lobe orifice (Fig 10.5). If manipulation of the tube is necessary, the tracheal lumen should be rechecked. It is also advisable to repeat the procedure after the

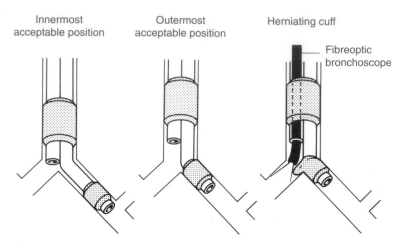

Figure 10.4   Left-sided double-lumen tube position. (After Aitkenhead AR, Jones RM. Clinical anaesthesia. Edinburgh: Churchill Livingstone; 1996, with permission.)

patient has been positioned for surgery. Despite accurate initial placement of endobronchial tubes, movement can occur during surgery, and repositioning can be difficult. It is useful to note the length of the tube at the teeth when it is first placed because this can be used later to estimate whether the tube has slipped in or out of the main bronchus.

Bronchial blockade

Bronchial blockers have been used intraoperatively for many years to block off individual lobes and facilitate OLV. There has been renewed interest in using bronchial blockade which has led to the development of a combined endotracheal tube and bronchial blocker, the Univent tube, and the availability of single endobronchial blockers.

The Univent tube

The Univent tube comprises an endotracheal tube with a moveable bronchial blocker attached (Fig 10.6).

    The tracheal tube has a small channel through the anterior internal wall which holds a bronchial blocker with a low pressure, high-volume cuff. The tube is placed in the trachea in the usual way and the blocker advanced, preferably under FOB control, to block the appropriate main or lobar bronchus. The blocker is then locked in place (Table 10.6).

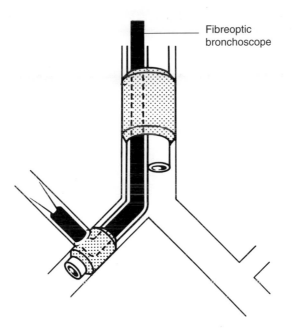

Fibreoptic
bronchoscope

Figure 10.5 Right-sided double-lumen tube in position. (After Aitkenhead AR, Jones RM. Clinical anaesthesia. Edinburgh: Churchill Livingstone; 1996, with permission.)

Table 10.6   Univent tube

Advantages	Disadvantages
Lobar blockade possible	Less versatile than double-lumen tube, problem with pneumonectomy
Ease of use for difficult intubation	Inflation/deflation of the lung more difficult
Facilitates aspiration of secretions	Blocker can migrate
No tube exchange if ventilation continued postoperatively	More expensive than double-lumen tube

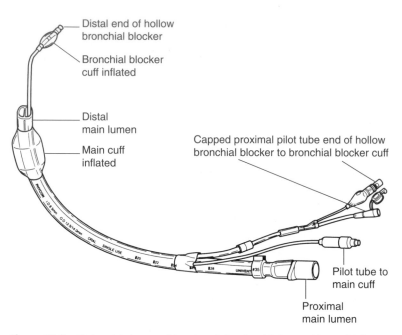

Distal end of hollow
bronchial blocker

Bronchial blocker
cuff inflated

Distal
main lumen

Main cuff
inflated

Capped proximal pilot tube end of hollow
bronchial blocker to bronchial blocker cuff

Pilot tube to
main cuff

Proximal
main lumen

Figure 10.6   Univent tube-combined endotracheal tube and bronchial
blocker. (After Gothard J, Kelleher A. Essentials of cardiac and thoracic
anaesthesia. Oxford: Butterworth Heinemann; 1999, with permission.)

Ventilation during thoracotomy
*Physiological consequences of the lateral thoracotomy
position*
In the awake subject, there is little or no additional ventilation/
perfusion mismatch in the lateral position. The situation changes during
anaesthesia. In the spontaneously breathing subject, there is a reduction
in inspiratory muscle tone (particularly the diaphragm) and a decrease
in the volume of both lungs with a reduction in functional residual
capacity. The compliance of the non-dependent upper lung increases
and it receives more ventilation. Paralysis and intermittent positive
pressure ventilation are used during thoracotomy and the compliance of
the non-dependent lung is increased even further. In practice, it is usual
to selectively ventilate the lower lung (OLV) at this point and allow the
upper lung to collapse. This eliminates the preferential ventilation and
facilitates surgical access, but creates the more serious problem of
ventilation/perfusion mismatch.

Physiology of one-lung anaesthesia
Venous admixture
Pulmonary blood flow continues to the upper lung during one-lung anaesthesia, creating a true shunt in a lung where there is blood flow to the alveoli but no ventilation. This shunt is the major cause of hypoxaemia during OLV, although the alveoli with low ventilation/perfusion ratios in the dependent lung also contribute. In addition, the blood to the upper lung cannot take up oxygen and therefore retains its poorly oxygenated mixed venous composition. This mixes with oxygenated blood in the left atrium causing venous admixture and lowering arterial oxygen tension (PaO_2). Total venous admixture can be calculated from the shunt equation which estimates what proportion of the pulmonary blood flow would have bypassed ventilated alveoli to produce the arterial blood gas values for a particular patient. Venous admixture and shunt (Qs/Qt) are often used synonymously.

Venous admixture increases from a value of approximately 10% to 15% during two lung ventilation to 30% to 40% during OLV. The PaO_2 can be maintained in the range of 9–16 kPa with an inspired oxygen concentration between 50% and 100% in the majority of patients.

Hypoxic pulmonary vasoconstriction and one-lung ventilation
Hypoxic pulmonary vasocontriction (HPV) is a mechanism whereby pulmonary blood flow is diverted away from hypoxic/collapsed areas of lung. This should improve oxygenation during OLV. Volatile anaesthetic agents depress HPV directly, but also enhance HPV by reducing cardiac output. There is therefore no change in the HPV response with volatile agents during thoracotomy and OLV.

Intravenous agents, such as propofol, do not inhibit HPV and should improve arterial oxygenation during OLV. There is some evidence to support this contention.

Cardiac output
Changes in cardiac output affect arterial oxygenation during thoracotomy. A decrease in cardiac output results in a reduced mixed venous oxygen content. Some of this desaturated blood is shunted during OLV and further exacerbates arterial hypoxaemia. Cardiac output can decrease for a number of reasons during thoracotomy. These include blood loss/fluid depletion, the use of high inflation pressures and the application of positive end-expiratory pressure (PEEP) to the dependent lung.

Surgical manipulation and retraction around the mediastinum, causing a reduction in venous return, are probably the commonest causes of a sudden drop in cardiac output during lung resection.

Principles of ventilation (Table 10.7)
OLV should be established to adequately inflate the lung but also minimize intra-alveolar pressure and so prevent diversion of pulmonary blood flow to the upper lung. In practice, this is not easy to achieve. It is reasonable to use an inspired oxygen concentration of 50% initially, which can be increased to 100%, if required. This cannot affect the true shunt in the upper lung but improves oxygenation through the alveoll with low V/Q ratios in the lower lung.

Overinflating the single lung ('volutrauma') can be detrimental and lead to acute lung injury. Deflation and inflation of the operative lung with the potential for ischaemia/reperfusion injury has also been implicated in lung damage. The use of low tidal volumes improves outcome in ventilated patients with adult respiratory distress syndrome and this may also apply to OLV. Limiting ventilation can lead to carbon dioxide retention, but a degree of permissive hypercapnia is preferable to lung trauma.

Hypoxia during one-lung ventilation
It is difficult to predict which patients are likely to be hypoxic (SpO$_2$ < 90%) during OLV. Patients with poor lung function are sometimes accepted for lung resection on the basis that their diseased lung is contributing little to gas exchange and this can be confirmed by V/Q scanning. Conversely, patients with normal lung function are more likely to be hypoxic during OLV because an essentially normal lung is collapsed to

---

Table 10.7   Guidelines for managing one-lung ventilation

Inspired oxygen concentration of 50% to 100%
    Increase if SpO$_2$ < 90%
Normal inspired/expired ratio (1 : 2)
    Increase expiratory phase if gas trapping likely
Consider pressure limiting ventilation
Use small tidal volumes (e.g. 6–7 ml/kg)
Allow permissive hypercapnia
Use positive end-expiratory pressure in hypoxic patients
Avoid overinflation ('volutrauma')

provide surgical access. The most significant predictors of a low arterial oxygen saturation during OLV are (1) a right-sided operation, (2) a low oxygen saturation during two-lung ventilation prior to OLV and (3) a high (or more normal) forced expiratory volume in 1 s preoperatively.

Once hypoxia occurs, it is important to check the position of the endobronchial tube and readjust this if necessary. A high inflation pressure (> 30–35 cmH_2O) may indicate that the tube is displaced. It may be helpful to analyse a flow/volume loop or at least manually reinflate the lung to feel the compliance. If a tube is obstructing a lobar orifice, only one or two lobes are being ventilated at most and hypoxia is likely. Suction and manual reinflation of the dependent lung may be useful.

Other measures which can be used to improve oxygenation include increasing the inspired oxygen concentration, introducing PEEP to the dependent lung, or supplying oxygen to the upper lung by via a continuous positive airway system, thereby reducing the shunt.

In the face of persistent arterial hypoxaemia during OLV, it is pertinent to ask 'What is a low PaO_2 for this patient?'. An oxygen saturation below 90% is commonly used. This arbitrary figure is affected by a variety of factors, including acidosis and temperature. Many patients will have a low PaO_2 when measured breathing air preoperatively; hence, the usefulness of this preoperative measurement. Arterial hypoxaemia is obviously undesirable but it may be preferable to accept a PaO_2 slightly lower than the preoperative value, rather than undertake measures such as upper lung inflation which may hinder and prolong surgery.

High-frequency jet ventilation

High-frequency jet ventilation (HFJV) can be used to provide satisfactory gas exchange during thoracotomy either by an endotracheal tube or some form of endobronchial tube. HFJV provides satisfactory ventilation by either route and has the advantage of low peak airway pressures, albeit with the production of obligatory PEEP by the majority of systems. Some clinicians advocate the use of HFJV during thoracic surgery and use it routinely. This method of ventilation has not been adopted widely as a result of difficulties with surgical access because the lung is distended and gaseous anaesthetic agents cannot be administered.

New modalities and one-lung anaesthesia

Ventilation, is the main area in which changes are made to reduce hypoxia during OLV. Increasing interest is shown in the pharmacological manipulation of pulmonary blood flow during OLV with prostaglandin E_1 and nitric oxide.

Termination of surgery and anaesthesia

Testing of bronchial suture lines

On completion of lung resection, the bronchial suture lines and lung surfaces are tested for an air leak. Sterile water is instilled into the pleural cavity, following cancer surgery, to cover the bronchial suture lines. After lobectomy, the remaining lobe or lobes are then suctioned before reinflation. In the case of pneumonectomy, very gentle suction is applied with a soft catheter to the bronchial stump. At this stage, it may be helpful to deflate the bronchial cuff. The bronchial stump is then tested for a leak as a positive pressure of approximately 25 cmH_2O is applied manually in a sustained manner to both lumina of the DLT.

In the unlikely event of a leak being present, gas bubbles will be seen appearing below the water level in the pleural cavity, indicating the need for further surgery. Testing for lung surface leaks is undertaken at a lower inflation pressure of approximately 20 cmH_2O.

Termination of anaesthesia

After completion of lung resection and closure of the chest wall, anaesthesia is lightened and spontaneous ventilation re-established in the usual manner. Before removal of the endobronchial tube, the patient is placed in a supine position. Following lobectomy, tracheobronchial suction is carried out to clear secretions and blood in the bronchi of the intact lung and the remaining lobes of the operated lung. The lungs are then manually reinflated again, also at a low pressure, with the chest drains open to an underwater seal drain. The endobronchial tube is removed when the patient's respiratory effort is satisfactory.

A similar sequence is followed after pneumonectomy but the remaining lung is reinflated until the trachea is approximately central, or slightly towards the side of surgery. The chest drain, if inserted, is then clamped. If a chest drain has not been used after pneumonectomy, it may be necessary to aspirate air from the hemithorax on the side of surgery to optimize the position of the mediastinum.

Patients are placed in the sitting position after removal of the DLT and allowed to breathe oxygen-enriched air. Further postoperative care is supervised in a high-dependency or intensive care unit.

Further reading

Aitkenhead AR, Jones RM (eds). Clinical anaesthesia. Edinburgh: Churchill Livingstone; 1996.

Brodsky JB, Benumof JL, Ehrenwerth J, Ozaki GT. Depth of placement of left double-lumen endobronchial tubes. Anesth Analg 1991;73:570–572.

Brodsky JB, Macario A, Mark BD. Tracheal diameter predicts double-lumen tube size: a method for selecting left double-lumen tubes. Anesth Analg 1996;82:861–864.

Chen TL, Lee YT, Wang MJ, Lee JM, Lee YC, Chu SH. Endothelin-1 concentrations and optimisation of arterial oxygenation by selective pulmonary artery infusion of prostaglandin E₁ during thoracotomy. Anaesthesia 1996;51:422–426.

Cohen E. Methods of lung separation. Curr Opin Anaesthesiol 2002;15:69–78.

Gosh S, Latimer RD. Thoracic anaesthesia: principles and practice. Oxford: Butterworth Heinemann; 1999.

Gothard JWW. Anaesthesia for thoracic surgery, 2nd edn. Oxford: Blackwell Scientific Publications; 1993.

Inoue H, Shotsu A, Ogawa J, Kawada S, Koide S. New device for one-lung anaesthesia: endotracheal tube with movable blocker. J Thorac Cardiovasc Surg 1982;83:940–941.

Kellow NH, Scott AD, White SA, Feneck RO. Comparison of the effects of propofol and isoflurane anaesthesia on right ventricular function and shunt fraction during thoracic surgery. Br J Anaesth 1995;75:578–582.

Nunn JF. Applied respiratory physiology, 4th edn. London: Butterworth Heinemann; 1993.

Reid CW, Slinger PD, Lenis S. A comparison of the effects of propofol-alfentanil anesthesia on arterial oxygenation during one-lung ventilation. J Cardiothorac Vasc Anesth 1996;10:860–863.

Robertshaw FL. Low resistance double-lumen endobronchial tubes. Br J Anaesth 1962;34:576–579.

Tugrul M, Camci E, Karadeniz H, Senturk M, Pembeci K, Akpir K. Comparison of volume controlled with pressure controlled ventilation during one-lung anaesthesia. Br J Anaesth 1997;79:306–310.

Williams EA, Evans TW, Goldstraw P. Acute lung injury following lung resection: is one lung anaesthesia to blame? Thorax 1996;51:114–116.

Wilson WC, Kapelanski DP, Benumof JL, Johson FW, Channick RN. Inhaled nitric oxide (40 ppm) during one-lung ventilation, in the lateral decubitus position does not decrease pulmonary vascular resistance or improve oxygenation in normal patients. J Cardiothorac Vasc Anesth 1997;11:172–176.

11

Intraoperative management of specific thoracic procedures

Bronchoscopy

Indications

Isolated rigid bronchoscopy has largely been superseded by flexible fibreoptic bronchoscopy for the initial diagnosis of lung and airway disease. Fibreoptic bronchoscopy is usually carried out by respiratory physicians under local anaesthesia, but rigid bronchoscopy remains the procedure of choice for surgical assessment of the airway before staging procedures such as mediastinotomy, or before lung resection. The rigid bronchoscope is also preferred for procedures such as removal of foreign bodies, stent insertion and resection of airway tumour. Current practice is summarized below.

Patient characteristics

All patients undergoing thoracotomy are bronchoscoped before surgery. Patients with lung cancer are often elderly smokers and their pre-operative evaluation has been dealt with in previous chapters. Patients may also present primarily with airway pathology and they will undergo rigid bronchoscopy as an isolated procedure, unless this is combined with a therapeutic procedure, such as dilatation of the trachea, resection of tumour or stent insertion.

Risk factors and preoperative assessment

For isolated bronchoscopy and therapeutic procedures, it is important to evaluate the upper airway and assess whether there is any clinical evidence of obstruction. Examination of the patient may reveal whether this obstruction is severe; for example, if there is breathlessness at rest, audible stridor or use of the accessory muscles of respiration. The following investigations may also be useful in defining the degree of obstruction before anaesthesia:

- Lung function tests (particularly the flow/volume loop).
- Chest X-ray – with additional lateral view of the trachea.
- Computed tomography or magnetic resonance imaging showing main airways.

Rigid bronchoscopy may entail a degree of neck extension which is particularly hazardous in the anaesthetized and paralysed patient. A lateral neck X-ray should be checked for abnormalities in patients with rheumatoid arthritis or a history of neck problems.

Monitoring/vascular access
- Peripheral venous access.
- Electrocardiogram (ECG).
- Pulse oximetry.
- Non-invasive blood pressure measurement.

Direct measurement of intra-arterial blood pressure is indicated in patients with severe upper airway obstruction.

Positioning
Rigid bronchoscopy is carried out with the patient in a supine position. The eyes should be protected and any vulnerable teeth or bridgework noted. The head is initially placed in a neutral position with one soft pillow in place. As the bronchoscope is advanced, it may be necessary to extend the neck and this can be carried out by carefully moving the head-end of the operating table down.

Airway and ventilatory management
The airway is 'shared' by the surgeon and anaesthetist throughout the whole procedure. The two main methods of providing gas exchange during rigid bronchoscopy are described below.

Venturi injector
A high pressure source of oxygen is intermittently injected through a fine needle at the proximal end of the bronchoscope creating a Venturi effect. Air is entrained and positive pressure produced at the distal end of the bronchoscope. Intermittent inflation/deflation provides satisfactory oxygenation and carbon dioxide clearance. The injector is usually controlled manually, although automatic control devices have

been described. It is essential to ensure there is an adequate opening at the proximal end of the bronchoscope to allow entrainment of air and, most importantly, if barotrauma is to be avoided, egress of gas during expiration. It is also important to match the injector needle size to the type of bronchoscope and oxygen pressure used (Table 11.1). This mode of ventilation is usually used in adults.

Table 11.1 Maximum inflation pressure achieved with various Venturi injector systems

Negus bronchoscope	Injector needle	Maximum pressure (cmH$_2$O)
Adult	14	50
Adult	16	25–30
Child	19	14–18
Suckling	18	15

Note: Adult Negus is equivalent to Adult Storz. Manual ventilation via a T piece is preferred with paediatric Storz bronchoscopes.

Ventilating bronchoscope

A glass slide device at the proximal end of the rigid bronchoscope allows manual positive-pressure ventilation with a suitable gas mixture via a side port built into the bronchoscope (Storz type). A rubber diaphragm can replace the glass window so that a telescope can be used down the bronchoscope whilst ventilation is continued. This technique is ideal for use in infants and children. A T piece circuit is attached to the side port of the bronchoscope and anaesthesia is maintained with gaseous agents and minimal risk of barotrauma.

Anaesthetic technique

Anaesthesia for rigid bronchoscopy should provide the following conditions: unconsciousness, muscular relaxation, abolition of respiratory tract reflexes, ventilation and a rapid recovery. A suitable anaesthetic technique for a short isolated bronchoscopy comprises:

• Light benzodiazepine premedication (omit with airway obstruction).
• Anti-sialogogue (use intravenous glycopyrrolate as necessary intraoperatively).
• Intravenous induction (propofol).

- Short-acting muscle relaxant (mivacurium or suxamethonium).
- Inhalational induction preferable in children and with upper airway obstruction.

Some anaesthetists elect to spray the vocal cords with plain lidocaine (maximum of 4 ml of 4%) before bronchoscopy to minimize post-operative laryngospasm.

Maintenance of anaesthesia is usually with intermittent bolus doses of an intravenous agent such as propofol. Awareness is a potential (and not uncommon) complication of bronchoscopy (Table 11.2). The incidence of myocardial ischaemia may be as high as 10% to 15% during bronchoscopy. The addition of remifentanil may improve haemo-dynamic stability. If bronchoscopy is prolonged, or is to be followed by a surgical procedure, a longer acting muscle relaxant such as vecuro-nium, or atracurium, can be given. Anaesthesia is then maintained with an infusion of propofol.

Postoperative management/complications

Muscular relaxation is reversed if necessary, and the patient allowed to awaken. Oxygen is administered by face mask and the patient is nursed in the lateral position with the diseased side down.

If there are no secretions or blood, the patient is nursed in the sitting position. Acute airway obstruction at this stage due to laryngospasm, presence of secretions or fragments of tumour is rare.

Table 11.2   Potential complications of bronchoscopy

- Damage to teeth
- Nasal bleeding (fibreoptic bronchoscopy)
- Aspiration of blood
- Awareness
- Pharyngeal rupture
    Mediastinitis
    Surgical emphysema
- Airway rupture/laceration
    Pneumothorax (? tension)
    Tracheo-oesophageal fistula
    Surgical emphysema
- Cardiac arrhythmias
- Hypertension
- Myocardial ischaemia
- Airway fires (laser)

Complex tracheal and endobronchial interventions
Bronchoscopy is required for more difficult procedures, such as tracheo-bronchial stent insertion, diathermy resection of tumours and laser therapy.

There is a considerable fire hazard when lasers are used in the presence of conventional tracheal tubes, particularly with a high oxygen concentration. Foil wrapped, or even metal, tracheal tubes have been used to provide an airway for laser treatment, but a simpler approach is to use a metal rigid bronchoscope for tracheal and endobronchial tumour resection.

The principles of bronchoscopy, as described above, can be applied to stent insertion procedures and resection of endobronchial tumour.

Removal of foreign bodies from the airway
Indications
All foreign bodies should be removed from the tracheobronchial tree. Acute upper airway obstruction is the immediate hazard when foreign bodies are inhaled but they often pass deeper into the tracheobronchial tree. Here, they impact and set up a local inflammatory reaction causing distal collapse and infection in the obstructed portion of lung.

Peanuts are commonly inhaled by small children and these swell *in situ*, fragment and liberate an irritant oil which causes severe local inflammation.

Patient characteristics
Foreign bodies are inhaled at any age but, most commonly, by children under the age of 3 years. A specific history of inhalation may be available, but this is often absent in children. Paroxysmal cough and wheeze are common presenting symptoms in children but dyspnoea, stridor and fever may also occur. A persistent chest infection which fails to clear after appropriate antibiotic therapy may warrant diagnostic bronchoscopy to exclude a foreign body in children. A chest X-ray (with inspiratory and expiratory films) may reveal obstructive emphysema with the foreign body acting as a ball-valve in a main bronchus. More often, radiological appearances are non-specific, with atelectasis and consolidation.

Risk factors and preoperative assessment
The immediate risk of foreign body inhalation is upper airway obstruction. This is unusual, but likely to be evident clinically. Premedication is often omitted in this group of patients.

Monitoring/vascular access
• As for bronchoscopy.

Airway and ventilatory management
Venturi ventilation is satisfactory for adults, but care must be taken not to blow the foreign body deeper into the tracheobronchial tree. The ventilating bronchoscope is preferable in children.

Anaesthetic technique
In adults, the anaesthetic techniques described for bronchoscopy are satisfactory in the majority of cases. An inhalational induction may be indicated in the presence of upper airway obstruction.

It is traditional to induce children with an inhalational agent. This has two advantages; first, cumulative doses of intravenous induction agent with delayed wakening, are avoided and, second, the airway can be safely maintained up to the time of bronchoscopy. Some anaesthetists continue with an inhalational agent to provide deep anaesthesia in the spontaneously breathing patient. A bronchoscope can then be inserted without muscle relaxation. We prefer an inhalational induction with sevoflurane followed by suxamethonium. Ventilation is then gently started via a T piece circuit connected to the ventilating bronchoscope. Anaesthesia can be maintained with either sevoflurane, or isoflurane, in a relatively high concentration of oxygen.

Muscle paralysis can be maintained with small incremental doses of suxamethonium, treating a bradycardia with intravenous atropine. If the procedure is prolonged, and there are no problems with ventilation, a non-depolarizing neuromuscular blocking drug is given.

Postoperative management/complications
After the foriegn body has been retrieved, anaesthesia is discontinued and any residual paralysis reversed. When the child is fully awake, spontaneous respiration can be allowed through the tube, and endotracheal suction carried out before extubation. Laryngeal stridor is relatively common at this time, particularly after a prolonged procedure in a small child. Intravenous dexamethasone and nebulized adrenaline may alleviate the problem. Reintubation, using an endotracheal tube smaller than would normally be chosen, is necessary if severe stridor or signs of respiratory obstruction are present. In extreme circumstances, a period of postoperative ventilation may be required.

Mediastinoscopy and mediastinotomy: diagnostic procedures

Indications

Mediastinoscopy is carried out with rigid mediastinoscope to provide a diagnosis in patients with mediastinal lymphadenopathy, and to assess operability in patients with lung cancer.

Anterior mediastinotomy, carried out through a small incision in the second interspace, allows exploration of tumours and lymph nodes of the anterior mediastinum which are inaccessible by mediastinoscopy. Left anterior mediastinotomy is used to assess the lymph node drainage of left upper lobe tumours visually, and also by digital palpation.

Patient characteristics

The majority of patients will have lung cancer.

Other indications for mediastinoscopy/mediastinotomy include hilar lymphadenopathy (sarcoidosis or malignant lymphadenopathy) and mediastinal tumours. Anterior mediastinal tumours can compromise the airway at tracheal or bronchial level and cause superior vena caval obstruction or even pulmonary artery obstruction. These patients are in a very high risk category. Thymic tumours may prove a problem because of associated myasthenia gravis. Rarely, a patient presenting for mediastinal biopsy will have the myasthenic syndrome.

Myasthenic syndrome and myasthenia gravis

A myopathy, with features resembling myasthenia gravis, was reported in association with malignant disease by Eaton and Lambert in the 1950s. Myasthenic syndrome is usually associated with small cell carcinoma of the bronchus, but occurs with other neoplasms. The myasthenic syndrome and myasthenia gravis are compared in Table 11.3.

The majority of patients with small cell cancer are inoperable and rarely undergo lung resection. However, they may present for bronchoscopy and mediastinoscopy. An effort should be made to avoid muscle relaxants.

If a conventional dose of muscle relaxant is given to a patient with the myasthenic syndrome, either inadvertently or because the condition has not been formally diagnosed, it is safer to ventilate the patient post-operatively and wait for the effect to wear off.

Risk factors: medistinoscopy and mediastinotomy

The main risk factors relate to the preoperative condition of the patient. The most significant intraoperative complication is major

Table 11.3   Features of myasthenia gravis and the myasthenic syndrome

Myasthenic syndrome	Myasthenia gravis
Clinical features	
Occurs mainly in elderly men. There is weakness and fatiguability of proximal limb muscles. Tendon reflexes are reduced or absent	More common in young women Initial muscle weakness usually in ocular, oropharyngeal and limb muscles
Response to muscle relaxants	
Sensitivity to both non-depolarizing and depolarizing drugs	Sensitive to non-depolarizing drugs Resistant to depolarizing drugs
Anticholinesterase therapy	
Poor response	Good response
Pathological features	
Associated with small cell carcinoma of the lung	Thymoma present in 20% to 25% of cases

bleeding, often related to inadvertent biopsy of a major vascular structure.

Monitoring/vascular access
- Peripheral venous access.
- ECG.
- Pulse oximetry.
- Non-invasive blood pressure measurement.

Positioning
For supine positioning, a sand bag is placed under the patient's shoulders, and the head, placed in a head ring, is extended as far back as safety permits. A slight head-up tilt prevents venous engorgement in the few patients with superior vena caval obstruction.

Airway and ventilatory management
Mediastinoscopy and mediastinotomy usually follow rigid broncho-scopy. After the bronchoscope is removed, a standard endotracheal tube is inserted and intermittent positive-pressure ventilation (IPPV) continued throughout the procedure.

Anaesthetic technique

Paralysis is maintained with a short acting non-depolarizing agent such as atracurium or vecuronium. Anaesthesia is continued with a suitable inhalational agent; nitrous oxide is avoided if pneumothorax is a potential hazard. Postoperative pain may be a problem following mediastinotomy, particularly if a section of costal cartilage has been excised.

During mediastinotomy, the pleura may be opened and this is drained during surgical closure. A large nasogastric tube is placed in the pleural space through the surgical incision and the lung is then expanded manually by the anaesthetist. As the muscle suture line is near completion, a sustained inflation pressure is applied to the lung, the tube is withdrawn, and the suture line completed.

Postoperative management/complications

At the end of mediastinoscopy or mediastinotomy, muscular relaxation is reversed in the usual manner and spontaneous respiration re-established. The endotracheal tube is removed after tracheobronchial suction and the patient returned to a recovery area breathing supplementary oxygen in a sitting position.

Surgery and the lung

Lobectomy and pneumonectomy

Chapters 9, 10 and 12 describe the anaesthetic and postoperative management of patients undergoing lung resection for lung cancer. These principles of management can be applied, with certain modifications, to patients undergoing lung resection for other pathology.

Lobectomy

Indications
- Malignant and benign tumours.
- Infection: bronchiectasis.
- Tuberculosis and fungal infection.

Patient characteristics
If the lobectomy is for primary lung cancer, the patients are likely to be elderly smokers. Lobectomy for benign tumour is uncommon. Excision of metastases requiring lobectomy is also likely to be in a younger age group. Lobectomy for bronchiectasis is uncommon, but is indicated if the disease is severely debilitating and confined to one or two lobes. Fungal infection (aspergilloma) is a rare indication for lobectomy.

Risk factors
These relate to the underlying pathology. Patients with bronchiectasis are admitted several days preoperatively for physiotherapy, postural drainage and antibiotic therapy.

Monitoring/vascular access
Together with anaesthetic technique and postoperative management, this is described further in Chapter 10.

Positioning
Lobectomy is carried out with the patient in a lateral position and the operative side uppermost.

Airway and ventilatory management
A double-lumen endobronchial tube is placed in the non-operative lung for lobectomy. One-lung ventilation (OLV) facilitates surgery but, at times, the surgeon may request reinflation of the upper lung whilst fissures are defined and dissected. In bronchiectasis, the remaining lobe or lobes on the operative side are unprotected from the spread of secretions if a double-lumen tube is used. In addition, infected secretions can seep past the endobronchial cuff into the opposite, dependent, lung. Repeated suction to both lungs limits this contamination.

Spread of secretions from lobe to lobe can be reduced by using bronchial blockade (e.g. Univent) to block specific bronchi whilst continuing to ventilate the remaining lobes.

Pneumonectomy
The usual indication for pneumonectomy is primary carcinoma of the lung. Anaesthesia and postoperative management for this procedure are discussed in Chapter 10

Occasionally, pneumonectomy is undertaken for other problems such as infection, or a 'completion pneumonectomy' may be carried out if there is recurrence of tumour after a previous lobectomy, or even a second primary. If pneumonectomy is undertaken for infection, it is usually because the lung has been totally destroyed by radiotherapy or tuberculosis. A pleuropneumonectomy is undertaken to contain spread of infection. and can result in significant blood loss. It is essential to isolate the remaining 'good' lung and a period of postoperative ventilation may be required.

Bronchopleural fistula

A bronchopleural fistula (BPF) is a direct communication between the tracheobronchial tree and the pleural cavity. Causes of BPF are listed in Table 11.4.

Minor forms of post-pneumonectomy BPF can be cauterized at bronchoscopy with sodium hydroxide, or may be sealed with a tissue glue. Large fistulas require surgical repair (resuture of the bronchial stump) via a lateral thoracotomy through the previous incision. The rate of BPF is < 1% after pneumonectomy. Occasionally, patients with chronic fistulae for repair are referred from other centres. They need sterilization of the pneumonectomy space and then the fistula is closed surgically. The principles of anaesthetic management are similar to those described below for an acute BPF. The surgery is more complicated, because muscle flaps, or omentum, are placed in the chest to obliterate the space around the repaired fistula. This may also be combined with a limited thoracoplasty.

Patient characteristics

Patients are often post-pneumonectomy (3–15 days) and ASA status IV or V. Rupture of the major airways after trauma is a form of BPF, which requires surgical repair.

Preoperative assessment

Symptoms relate to infected, pneumonectomy-space fluid flowing in to the remaining lung. This leads to malaise, low grade fever, cough with wheeze and dyspnoea. Acute onset of a large BPF presents with severe dyspnoea and the patient coughing up large amounts of brownish, infected, space fluid.

Table 11.4   Causes of bronchopleural fistula

- Dehiscence of bronchial stump after lung resection
    Lobectomy
    Pneumonectomy (most common: right > left)
- Trauma
    Rupture of main bronchi
        Deceleration injury
        Usually within 2–2.5 cm of the carina
- Neoplasm
- Inflammatory lesions
    Tuberculosis

A chest X-ray usually confirms the diagnosis showing a loss of pneu-monectomy space fluid and collapse/consolidation, or increased shad-owing, in the remaining lung. With a smaller chronic fistula, the chest X-ray may only show a slght drop in the level of the space fluid.

Initial treatment

The patient is resuscitated, given oxygen and an intravenous infusion started. Most importantly, the patient should be sat upright to prevent further spillover and a chest drain inserted on the pneumonectomy side to remove remaining fluid (no suction should be applied). The patient should be moved to theatre in a sitting position with the drain unclamped, but with the underwater seal bottle below the bed or trolley.

Monitoring/vascular access

For major thoracic surgery (Chapter 10, Table 10.2).

- Place arterial line before induction.

Anaesthetic technique/airway management

Classically, it has been assumed that a post-pneumonectomy BPF should be isolated by means of an endobronchial tube placed in the remaining lung before IPPV is employed. A double-lumen tube is inserted therefore in the remaining bronchus. To secure the airway before administration of a muscle relaxant, two methods were *previously* advocated:

- Awake endobronchial intubation using local analgesia of the upper respiratory tract.
- Inhalational induction and intubation under deep inhalational anaesthesia.

Both techniques are fraught with difficulty, particularly in these debili-tated patients. The following technique is now used to anaesthetize a patient with an acute BPF:

- Patient sitting upright with drain open.
- Keep in semi-sitting position, if possible.
- Monitoring as detailed above.
- Preoxygenation.
- Slow intravenous induction.
- Intravenous suxamethonium.

- Insertion of double-lumen tube (preferably under direct vision with fibreoptic bronchoscope).
- Administer non-depolarizing muscle relaxant once lung isolated.
- IPPV via endobronchial portion of the tube.
- Place patient in the lateral position for thoracotomy.

Postoperative management

Re-establishment of spontaneous respiration in the sitting position is ideal because it protects the repaired bronchial stump from positive-pressure ventilation. In practice, respiratory failure is common after this procedure and it should be managed conventionally with IPPV through an endotracheal tube. High-frequency jet ventilation has been advocated because of the low peak airway pressure generated.

Mortality is high following repair of post-pneumonectomy BPF.

Video-assisted thoracoscopic surgery

Video-assisted thoracoscopic surgery (VATS) has been widely adopted for pleurectomy, lung biopsy, drainage of effusions/talc pleurodesis and lung volume reduction surgery (Table 9.1).

VATS is considered less invasive than open thoracotomy and can be carried out through a series of ports inserted through the chest wall. Postoperative pain is less than after open thoracotomy and length of hospital stay decreased.

Anaesthetic considerations for video-assisted thoracoscopic surgery

Anaesthetic techniques for VATS are little different from those employed for lung resection.

Lung collapse/deflation on the operative side is mandatory and can usually be achieved with a left-sided endobronchial tube because this type of surgery does not breach the airway. Nitrous oxide should be omitted from the inspired gas in those patients with a pneumothorax.

Lung collapse during OLV may be slow in the presence of marked emphysema and a variety of techniques have been used to promote this. Some centres insufflate carbon dioxide into the pleural cavity. Once the surgeons have visualized the space and divided adhesions, lung collapse is usually sufficient to allow definitive surgery to proceed.

OLV is managed as described for lung resection (see Chapter 10) for most VATS procedures. It is important with lung volume reduction surgery (LVRS) to limit inflation pressure and also increase the expiratory phase of ventilation.

Minor VATS procedures can be carried out without invasive arterial monitoring. Postoperative pain is not severe following VATS, except for pleurectomy, for which epidural analgesia may be used.

The majority of patients can be extubated in the usual way immediately following VATS procedures. Occasionally, patients may not be able to sustain spontaneous respiration initially.

Lung volume reduction surgery

There has been recently been a resurgence of interest in the surgical treatment of diffuse emphysema.

Indications

Patients selected for LVRS should have severe airflow obstruction mainly as a result of an emphysematous process (not primary airways disease). The emphysematous process should be regionally heterogeneous to provide 'target areas' for surgical resection and therefore leave less diseased lung tissue. These patients should also have marked thoracic hyperinflation and flattened diaphragms associated with air trapping. Predominant airways disease, hypercapnia and pulmonary hypertension are relative contraindications to surgery. Guidelines for patient selection and LVRS are shown in Table 11.5.

Mechanisms of improvement in lung function after lung volume reduction surgery

Reducing lung volume in diffuse emphysema improves elastic recoil of the lung. Airflow is also enhanced by increasing traction on the parenchymal airways and improved airway conductance. Lobectomy does not confer these important increases in airway conductance because of the simultaneous removal of conducting airways. Ventilatory mechanics can improve immediately following LVRS allowing early extubation. Additional benefits may include the recruitment of alveoli previously compressed by bullae and improved ventilation–perfusion matching because of enhanced right ventricular function.

Surgical approaches for lung volume reduction surgery

A variety of surgical techniques have been developed for LVRS. These include:

- Bilateral, stapling, lung volume reduction via a mediansternotomy.
- Laser therapy for bullous emphysema.
- VATS stapling LVRS.

Table 11.5   Guidelines for lung volume reduction surgery

Inclusion criteria
Patients on optimal medical therapy

Severe intractable breathlessness caused by emphysema/
  hyperinflation

Diagnosis of emphysema on computed tomography and chest X-ray
  (plus tests below)

Preferably heterogeneous disease with 'target areas'

Age < 75 years

Non-smoking (check urinary nicotine)

Able to understand risk/benefit

Spirometry and lung volumes
  Forced expiratory volume in 1 s < 35% predicted
  Residual volume > 250% predicted
  Residual volume/total lung capacity ratio > 60%

Cardiovascular function
  Normal right and left heart function

Exclusion criteria
Estimated life expectancy < 2 years

Spirometry and lung volumes
  Forced expiratory volume in 1 s > 50% predicted
  Residual volume < 150% predicted
  Total lung capacity < 100% predicted
  Forced expiratory volume in 1 s < 500 ml (Brompton Hospital)

Oxygen prescription > 18 h day

Hypercapnia (PaCO$_2$ > 6.0 kPa)

Corticosteroid requirement > 10 mg per day

Also:
  Previous thoracotomy
  Kyphoscoliosis
  Coronary artery disease
  Major medical disease other than emphysema

The VATS approach eliminates the complications of mediansternotomy.

VATS provides good access for lung volume reduction and better visualization of posterior and inferior adhesions than mediansternotomy. It can be carried out as a bilateral procedure. Routine chest drainage is employed.

Anaesthetic management of LVRS
The principles are summarized below:

Preoperative preparation
- All selected patients undergo an intensive rehabilitation and exercise programme.
- Medical treatment is optimized.

Premedication
- None.

Monitoring and vascular access
- As for major lung resection.

Induction and maintenance of anaesthesia
- Intravenous induction with propofol.
- Vecuronium or atracurium used as muscle relaxant.
- Maintenance on air/oxygen mixture with either isoflurane or propofol infusion.

Analgesia
It is essential to provide good postoperative analgesia; ideally, thoracic or lumbar epidural blockade with local anaesthetic agents alone or in combination with opioids.

Airway management
A left-sided, double-lumen tube is preferred for this type of surgery, its position should be checked by fibreoptic bronchoscopy.

Ventilation
The principles of management are:

- Keep the airway pressure low.
- Do not use positive end-expiratory pressure.
- Pressure limit to 20 cmH_2O on two lungs.
- Pressure limit to 30 cmH_2O on OLV.
- Allow permissive hypercapnia.
- Allow time for expiration (e.g. inspiratory : expiratory ratio 1 : 3 or longer).

If there are signs of air trapping, or hyperinflation of the ventilated lung, it is safer to transiently disconnect the patient from the ventilator to allow deflation. A period of gentle manual ventilation may be required thereafter. OLV may be particularly hazardous when the 'second' lung is being reduced during a bilateral procedure. Hypercapnia and hypoxia are common at this time.

Postoperative management
Early resumption of spontaneous respiration followed by rapid extubation is ideal. This should be possible with good analgesia.

The pleurae will be drained routinely but, despite meticulous surgery, air leaks are a major problem.

Surgery of the oesophagus
In general, many of the principles of anaesthesia for lung resection can be applied to oesophageal surgery. Preoperative assessment is similar, although there are specific features of oesophageal pathology, such as obstruction or the presence of a hiatus hernia, which are important. The principles of general anaesthesia, OLV and postoperative management for lung resection are equally applicable to major oesophageal surgery.

Surgery of the oesophagus in adults is mainly concerned with the management of reflux syndromes (i.e. hiatus hernia repair) and the treatment of oesophageal carcinoma. Surgery is carried out less frequently for other conditions such as benign stricture, diverticulum and achalasia of the oesophagus. Most patients will undergo oesophagoscopy before definitive surgery.

Reflux syndromes, hiatus hernia, achalasia
The cricopharyngeus muscle closes off the pharynx and acts as an upper oesophageal sphincter, but the lower oesophageal sphincter (LOS) is the major barrier preventing reflux from the stomach into the lower oesophagus.

The LOS is an area of circular muscle fibres 2–5 cm long innervated via the parasympathetic system. In normal subjects, the LOS extends above and below the diaphragm and its pressure increases in response to an elevation of intra-abdominal pressure, thereby maintaining a barrier between stomach and oesophagus. This mechanism fails in oesophageal abnormalities such as hiatus hernia. Induction of anaesthesia followed by the administration of muscle relaxants is particularly likely to lead to regurgitation of stomach contents in patients with LOS dysfunction, unless appropriate precautions are taken.

Achalasia of the oesophagus is a generalized disorder of oesophageal motility characterized by incoordinate or absent peristalsis. The LOS tone in these patients is normal or slightly elevated. The oesophagus gradually dilates, becomes grossly enlarged, and filled with food residues and secretions. These patients are at high risk from aspiration at induction of anaesthesia. They often suffer repeated episodes of aspiration before surgery which may result in bronchopneumonia and even lung abscess. The oesophagus is emptied via a rigid oesophagoscope before surgery.

Prevention of reflux at induction of anaesthesia is by a rapid sequence induction with cricoid pressure. Other measures taken to reduce gastric acid secretion and promote gastric emptying are summarized in Table 11.6.

Carcinoma of the oesophagus

Severe progressive dysphagia is the characteristic symptom of oesophageal carcinoma.

Table 11.6   Management of aspiration in oesophageal surgery

Drug therapy

Proton pump inhibitor
  Omeprazole, lansoprazole (or other suitable drug) the night before surgery

H_2 receptor antagonist
  Ranitidine, cimetidine (or other suitable alternative) the night before and 2 h before surgery
  Consider intravenous administration with dysphagia

Metoclopramide
  Stimulates gastric emptying and small intestinal transit, give with premedication

Antacids
  Sodium citrate (30 ml of an 0.3 molar solution) orally 30 min before surgery (clear fluid – does not obscure view at oesophagoscopy)

Physical methods
  Rapid sequence induction
  Cricoid pressure
  Slight head-up tilt

Patients presenting for oesophagoscopy and potentially oesopha-gectomy, may be dehydrated, debilitated and generally malnourished as a consequence of dysphagia. Anaemia and hypoalbuminaemia are common. In addition, many of these patients are elderly smokers and have cardiovascular and respiratory risk factors in common with lung resection patients. Oesophageal carcinoma is also associated with a high alcohol intake.

Efforts should be made to improve nutrition preoperatively, particu-larly if an extensive surgical resection is planned. A high calorie/high protein liquid diet may be tolerated if the oesophagus is not completely obstructed. Alternatively, a percutaneous endoscopic gastrostomy pro-vides a route for direct enteral feeding.

Oesophagoscopy
Indications
Oesophagoscopy is used for endoscopic examination and biopsy of tumours, removal of foreign bodies, dilatation of strictures and palli-ative intubation of malignant obstruction. A rigid oesophagoscope, inserted under general anaesthesia, gives a good view of the oeso-phageal mucosa and is large enough to allow the passage of large biopsy forceps and dilators.

The flexible fibreoptic oesophagoscope can be used with only topical analgesia and light sedation.

Risk factors
The main risk factors of this procedure are regurgitation/acid aspiration at induction of anaesthesia and concomitant medical disease.

Premedication
Oral premedication with temazepam is usually satisfactory. If the patient is debilitated, or has dysphagia, this can be omitted. Antacid prophylaxis is given, if appropriate.

Monitoring/vascular access
Monitoring requirements are similar to bronchoscopy with an ECG, non-invasive blood pressure measurement and pulse oximetry as a minimum. End-tidal gas analysis is also useful. Intraoperative arrhy-thmias are not uncommon, but are usually benign and do not require treatment.

Positioning

Oesophagoscopy is carried out with the patient in a supine position. If this is carried out on an operating table, the head can easily be extended to facilitate passage of the rigid oesophagoscope.

Anaesthetic technique/airway management

Induction

An intravenous induction with propofol is satisfactory in the majority of cases, but dosage should be kept to a minimum in elderly and/or debilitated patients. A rapid sequence induction, with the application of cricoid pressure, is undertaken in those patients at risk of aspiration.

Muscular relaxation

It is important to establish complete muscular relaxation so that the oesophagoscope can be safely passed through the cricopharyngeal sphincter. Suxamethonium is still the best drug if cricoid pressure is used, and this can be repeated in incremental doses for a short procedure. For a longer procedure, atracurium or mivacurium can be given.

Alternatively, these latter drugs can be given from the outset if there is no risk of aspiration.

Intubation

Endotracheal intubation is carried out with an armoured oral tube one size smaller than normal. The tracheal cuff may need to be deflated slightly to allow passage of the oesophagoscope through cricopharyngeus.

Maintenance of anaesthesia

Anaesthesia is usually maintained with an oxygen/air or an oxygen/nitrous oxide inspired gas mixture combined with a suitable inhalational agent. A propofol infusion is also satisfactory.

Post-operative management/complications

At the end of the procedure muscular relaxation is reversed, if necessary, and the patient extubated when awake in a lateral position.

A post-operative chest X-ray is mandatory for signs of oesophageal rupture, including surgical emphysema, pneumothorax, pneumomediastinum and pneumoperitoneum, before oral fluids are commenced.

Surgery for carcinoma of the oesophagus

Indications

The majority of tumours are in the middle and lower thirds of the oesophagus and can be resected via a left thoracoabdominal approach. Stomach or colon is then mobilized and brought up to restore the continuity of the alimentary tract. Oesophagogastrectomy may be required if the stomach is involved. Operative mortality remains high for these procedures and long-term survival depends on the extent of nodal spread at the time of surgery.

Although the left thoracoabdominal approach is popular, a variety of different surgical techniques may be used. The sequence of the planned procedure should be fully discussed with the surgeon before operation as this will have a major influence on positioning of the patient and the sites of vascular access.

Patient characteristics

These patients are often elderly smokers (male > female), with the additional systemic and metabolic consequences of dysphagia. The risk factors relate to the major nature of the surgery in a group of patients who may range from ASA status II–IV. The preoperative assessment of these patients is similar to that described for lung resection in Chapter 9. Postoperatively, anastomotic leaks are a major and significant source of morbidity and mortality, as are pulmonary and cardiovascular problems.

Premedication

- Light, oral, premedication is prescribed in the majority of patients.
- Antibiotic prophylaxis, commonly a cephalosporin and metronidazole, is started immediately after induction of anaesthesia.

Monitoring/vascular access

Monitoring and vascular access is as described for a major lung resection. If a high colonic or gastric anastomosis is planned via a cervical incision, central venous lines should not be sited in the neck.

Blood and fluid loss can be extensive during major oesophageal surgery. There is considerable heat loss during a thoracoabdominal laparotomy and a convective warm-air heating device is used to maintain body temperature.

Positioning

Positioning will depend entirely on the planned procedure. Commonly, a semilateral position is used.

Airway and ventilatory management

A double-lumen endobronchial tube is used to provide one-lung anaesthesia and facilitate surgical access to the oesophagus. A left-sided tube eliminates the problem of right upper lobe ventilation, but some surgeons prefer a right-sided tube for a left thoracoabdominal procedure. This is because a left-sided tube is more likely to kink and obstruct as the left lung is retracted to mobilize the oesophagus.

Deficiencies in the management of double-lumen tubes during OLV for oesophageal surgery were highlighted in the 1996/1997 National Confidential Enquiry into Perioperative Deaths. The management of endobronchial intubation is complex and should not be undertaken by the 'occasional' thoracic anaesthetist for complex oesophageal surgery.

Anaesthetic technique

An intravenous induction is used. Cricoid pressure is applied, where necessary, in which case suxamethonium is given as the initial muscle relaxant. Otherwise a non-depolarizing agent is used from the outset.

Epidural analgesia is extremely useful because of the pain produced by a large thoracoabdominal incision. This is established immediately after induction of anaesthesia in the high lumbar region.

Postoperative management

Early resumption of spontaneous respiration may be satisfactory, and even preferred, after a straightforward procedure with effective epidural analgesia. However, the endotracheal tube should only be removed when the patient is alert and in a sitting position. This is because a conduit of stomach or colon does not provide a mechanical barrier to prevent aspiration of gut/stomach contents.

A period of postoperative ventilation is usual in most patients.

Further reading

Aitkenhead AR. Anaesthesia for oesophageal surgery. In: Gothard JWW (ed.). Thoracic anaesthesia. Clinical Anaesthesiology, vol. 1. London: Baillière Tindall; 1987. pp. 181–206.

Baraka A. Anaesthesia and myasthenia gravis. Can J Anaesthesiol 1992; 39:476–486.

Boscoe MJ. Lung and heart-lung transplantation. In: Goldstone JC, Pollard BJ (eds). Handbook of clinical anaesthesia vol. 23. London: Churchill Livingstone; 1996. pp. 467–469.

Bracken CA, Gurkwoski MA, Naples JJ. Lung transplantation: historical perspective, current concepts, and anesthetic considerations. J Cardiothorac Vasc Anesth 1997;11:220–241.

Brenner M, Yusen R, McKenna R, Sciurba F, Gelb AF, Fischel R, Swain J, Chen JC, Kafie F, Lefrak SS. Lung volume reduction surgery for emphysema. Chest 1996;110:205–218.

Conacher I. Anaesthesia for the surgery of emphysema. Br J Anaesth 1997;79:530–538.

Cooper JD, Trulock EP, Triantafillou AN, Patterson GA, Pohl MS, Deloney PA, Sundaresan RS, Roper CL. Bilateral pneumectomy (volume reduction) for chronic obstructive pulmonary disease. J Thorac Cardiovasc Surg 1995;109:106–119.

Eaton LM, Lambert LM. Electromyography and electrical stimulation of nerves in disease with motor units. Observations on myasthenic syndrome associated with malignant tumours. JAMA 1957;163:1117–1124.

Eisenkraft JB. Myasthenia gravis and thymic surgery – anaesthetic considerations. In: Gothard JWW (ed.). Thoracic anaesthesia. Clinical anaesthesiology, vol. 1. London: Baillière Tindall; 1987. pp. 133–162.

Gold SJ, Duthie DJR. Anaesthesia for adult bronchoscopy. Bulletin 3. London: The Royal College of Anaesthetists; 2000.

Gothard JWW. Anaesthesia for thoracic malignancy. In: Filshie J, Robbie DS (eds). Anaesthesia and maligant disease. London: Edward Arnold; 1989.

Hill AJ, Feneck RO, Underwood SM, Davis ME, Marsh A, Bromley L. The haemodynamic effects of bronchoscopy. Comparison of propofol and thiopentone with and without alfentanil. Anaesthesia 1991;46:266–270.

Mentzelopoulos SD, Tzoufi MJ. Anesthesia for tracheal and endobronchial interventions. Curr Opin Anaesthesiol 2002;15:85–94.

Pfitzner J, Peacock MJ, Pfitzner L. Speed of collapse of the non-ventilated lung during one-lung anaesthesia: the effects of the use of nitrous oxide in sheep. Anaesthesia 2001;56:933–939.

Plummer S, Hartley M, Vaughan RS. Anaesthesia for telescopic procedures in the thorax. Br J Anaesth 1998;80:223–234.

Prakash N, McLeod T, Gao Smith F. The effects of remifentanil on haemodynamic stability during rigid bronchoscopy. Anaesthesia 2001;56:568–584.

Robertson R, Muers M. Mediastinal masses. Medicine 1995;23:369–371.

Sherry KM. How can we improve the outcome of oesophagectomy? (editorial.) Br J Anaesth 2001;86:611–613.

Tschernko EM, Wisser W, Hofer S, Kocher A, Watzinger U, Kritzinger M, Wislocki W, Klepetko W. The influence of lung volume reduction on ventilatory mechanics in patients suffering from severe chronic obstructive pulmonary disease. Anesth Analg 1996;83:996–1001.

Vanderschueren R. Pleural disease. Medicine 1995;23:256–261.

Walsh TS, Young CH. Anaesthesia and cystic fibrosis. Anaesthesia 1995;50:614–622.

Young-Beyer P, Wilson RS. Anesthetic management for tracheal resection and reconstruction. J Cardiothorac Anesth 1988;2:821–835.

12

Postoperative management: thoracic surgery

In the immediate postoperative period, the main concerns are to establish a satisfactory respiratory pattern, haemodynamic stability and good analgesia. This is best accomplished in a high-dependency unit (HDU). The majority of patients will be extubated in the operating theatre once spontaneous respiration has been established. However, some patients will require a period of mechanical ventilation.

The spontaneously breathing patient is nursed in the upright sitting position. Supplementary oxygen is supplied by face mask, preferably a fixed performance device. The invasive monitoring used in the operating theatre is continued in the HDU and rewarming completed with warm-air heating device. Initial investigations include arterial blood gas analysis, serum electrolytes, a full blood count and a chest X-ray. Clotting studies will be required if there is excess blood loss into the chest drains. Specific points to note in the first postoperative chest X-ray are shown in Table 12.1.

Respiratory management
Some patients may require a short period of mechanical ventilation while the effects of anaesthetic agents and opioids (intravenous or epidural) are allowed to 'wear off' rather than be abruptly antagonized with naloxone. These patients are ventilated through the double-lumen

---

Table 12.1   Specific points to note in initial postoperative chest X-ray

- Position of mediastinum
- Full expansion of lung fields
- Evidence of pneumothorax
- Position of endotracheal tube, if present
- Position of central venous lines
- Presence of pleural fluid

tube, with the bronchial cuff deflated and/or the tube partially withdrawn into the trachea.

Frail elderly patients with poor lung function, who have undergone extensive surgery, benefit from elective postoperative ventilation. In this group, the double-lumen tube is changed to an endotracheal tube at the end of surgery. Ventilation allows rewarming, correction of fluid/acid–base balance, optimum recovery from intraoperative atelectasis, and the establishment of adequate analgesia.

Intermittent positive-pressure ventilation is established and optimized in the usual manner. An attempt is made to keep inflation pressures within the normal range to protect the bronchial stump anastomosis.

Chest drainage

Pleural or chest drainage is an essential part of the management of the post-thoracotomy patient. Chest drains allow the escape of air, blood or fluid from the pleural space and restore cardiorespiratory function by re-expansion of the lung and elimination of mediastinal shift. The essential components of a simple chest drainage system are shown in Table 12.2.

Chest drainage after lung resection

Two chest drains are commonly inserted following lung resection (other than pneumonectomy). Classically, an apical drain is used to remove air which has risen towards the apex and a basal drain collects fluid which has gravitated downwards (Fig. 12.1). An alternative, and

---

Table 12.2   Components of a chest drainage system

- Pleural tube
    To evacuate air, blood or fluid with minimum resistance
    A 32-French gauge tube is commonly used (with -10 cmH$_2$O
        suction this will allow an airflow of approximately 35–40 l/min)
- Underwater seal
    One-way valve to allow expulsion of air and fluid and prevent
        re-entry of air on inspiration.
- Collecting chamber
    For blood/fluid
- Suction
    Usually 5 kPa
    Must be capable of clearing large volumes of air

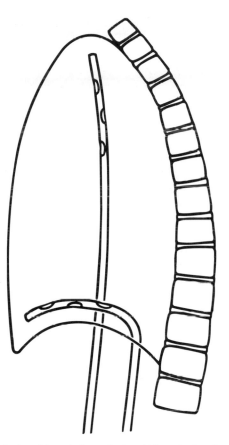

Figure 12.1   Apical and basal chest drains. (After Gothard J. Anaesthesia for thoracic surgery, 2nd edn. Oxford: Blackwell Scientific Publications; 1993, with permission.)

equally effective approach, is to place anterior and posterior drains towards the apex with side holes to provide basal drainage (Fig. 12.2).

Chest drainage after pneumonectomy

Air leak does not occur after pneumonectomy and chest drainage is not mandatory. Some surgeons, therefore, close the chest without a drain. If a chest drain is not inserted, air is aspirated from the pneumonectomy space at the end of operation, with the patient in a supine position. This can be performed simply with a 50-ml syringe and a three-way tap connected to a long intravenous cannula placed through the chest wall.

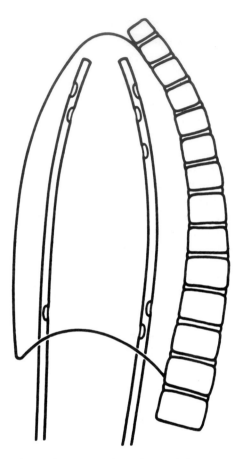

Figure 12.2   Anterior and posterior chest drains. (After Gothard J. Anaesthesia for thoracic surgery, 2nd edn. Oxford: Blackwell Scientific Publications; 1993, with permission.)

Several hundred millilitres of air are aspirated until there is a slight 'pull' on the syringe, indicating a negative pressure within the empty hemithorax. At this stage, the mediastinum, which will have moved towards the dependent lung during lateral thoracotomy, should be approximately central or slightly towards the side of surgery. This position can be verified crudely by feeling the position of the trachea or, more accurately, by inspecting the postoperative chest X-ray. Occasionally, it may be necessary to aspirate further air in the postoperative period.

Some surgeons prefer to place a chest drain in all patients following pneumonectomy, but particularly if there have been problems with bleeding. This is usually a single basal drain which is left clamped, but connected to an underwater seal drain. Traditionally, the clamp is released for 1–2 min every hour to show blood loss and centralize the mediastinum by releasing trapped air. Suction is *not* applied to a pneumonectomy drain under any circumstances. This will pull the mediastinum across and severely impede or totally obstruct venous return to the heart with disastrous consequences. Pneumonectomy drains are removed the day after surgery if there is no active bleeding.

Design of underwater seal drains

An underwater seal is essentially a one-way valve mechanism to allow expulsion of air and fluid out of the pleural space and to prevent re-entry of atmospheric air. Various designs of drainage bottle are made but, in theory, a large diameter bottle is preferable with the chest drain/connecting tube ending only 2 cm below the water surface (Fig. 12.3). This provides minimal resistance to the escape of air but a huge inspiratory effort would be required to break the seal by drawing water into the tubing from the bottle, providing the bottle is kept well below the patient. A large diameter collecting bottle is desirable so that the volume of water above the submerged drainage tubing is greater than the volume of the drainage tubing from patient to bottle.

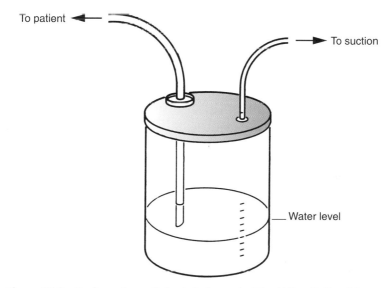

Figure 12.3   Underwater seal chest drainage bottle. (After Gothard J. Anaesthesia for thoracic surgery, 2nd edn. Oxford: Blackwell Scientific Publications; 1993, with permission.)

The main disadvantage of this simple system is the increasing resistance to drainage as the bottle fills with blood or fluid. This resistance to drainage is largely overcome by the use of suction.

Suction applied to chest drains

Suction increases the pressure difference between the pleural space and the chest drain bottle by drawing air from the bottle. Suction promotes expansion of the lung and assists the escape of air or fluid from the pleural space. It also eliminates the possibility of air entering the chest.

Low pressure suction (up to 5 kPa or 50 cmH$_2$O) may be applied but this must be provided by a pump capable of clearing large volumes of air. Modern pipeline low-pressure suction units are usually adequate in the face of all but the largest air leaks. Low pressure, low volume devices, such as the Roberts pump, cannot clear large volumes of air and may act as an obstruction to drainage in the presence of a large air leak.

Excessive or persistent air leak

The volume of air leak may, very rarely, be unacceptable in the immediate postoperative period and re-exploration is justified in case the lung has been transfixed by pericostal sutures. More commonly, the air leak will progressively lessen as the lung tissue expands to fill the thoracic cavity and seals the air leak against the chest wall.

Removal of chest drains

Chest drains are removed once they have ceased to function. This means when air or fluid loss has not occurred over the preceding 12–24 h and when the pleural space has been obliterated, as shown by the chest X-ray, the cessation of bubbling within the drainage bottle and the reduction of the respiratory swing of the water level.

There may be some discomfort during the removal of the drains and so a natural tendency for patients to inspire. Removal is undertaken during a Valsalva manoeuvre at full inspiration, thereby maintaining a positive intrapleural pressure and preventing influx of air. A horizontal mattress suture placed around the chest drain at the time of its insertion is tightened as the drain is removed to prevent air entering by the wound. After removal, a chest X-ray is obtained to exclude a pneumothorax.

Sputum retention

Sputum retention after thoracic surgery is common in smokers. Smoking induces mucus gland hyperplasia and mucosal metaplasia, together with impaired cilial function.

Patients with poor lung function, and particularly those whose forced expiratory volume in 1 s (FEV_1) < 1.0 l postoperatively, cannot cough effectively to clear secretions. In addition, damage to the recurrent laryngeal nerve and/or phrenic nerve reduces the force of coughing. Chest wall resection can cause a degree of paradoxical respiration, even after the insertion of a rigid chest wall prosthesis.

Physiotherapy, in the presence of adequate analgesia, is an effective method of clearing retained sputum.

If simple measures fail to solve the problem of sputum retention, a mini-tracheostomy tube can be inserted through the cricothyroid membrane as a direct route for bronchial suction. This procedure, carried out under local anaesthesia, is usually straightforward but, in unskilled hands, it can cause disaster. Continuing difficulties with sputum clearance can result in endotracheal intubation and mechanical ventilation. Formal tracheostomy may be required to aid weaning from ventilation in this small group of patients.

Respiratory failure

There is restricted ventilation and an altered pattern of breathing after thoracotomy. The characteristic mechanical abnormalities result in a reduction in vital capacity, tidal volume and FEV_1, as well as a decrease in functional residual capacity associated with anaesthesia.

Pain is the principal inhibitor of chest wall movement, but obesity, the supine position and interstitial oedema of damaged tissue all have a restrictive effect on ventilation. Postoperative hypoxaemia is almost inevitable following thoracotomy and is out of proportion to the quantity of lung removed or collapsed. Patients who are hypoxaemic preoperatively, not surprisingly, are more likely to be so postoperatively. Measures to minimize hypoxaemia and pulmonary complications are shown in Table 12.3.

Table 12.3   Measures to decrease pulmonary complications

- Provision of adequate analgesia
- Erect or semi-erect body position to increase functional residual capacity
- Humidified oxygen
- Regular physiotherapy
- Incentive spirometry
- Continuous positive pressure intermittently by face mask

Carbon dioxide retention is also a problem after thoracotomy. During the first few hours after surgery, hypercarbia is common. As satisfactory analgesia is established in the patient awakening from anaesthesia, serial blood gas analyses are undertaken. A raised $PaCO_2$ is not of great concern provided that the trend of serial estimations is downwards and the patient is awake with a satisfactory respiratory pattern. The patient is not transferred to a ward high dependency area until the $PaCO_2 \leq 7.0$ kPa. Chronic obstructive pulmonary disease is common in patients presenting for thoracic surgery, although this is unlikely to be severe in those scheduled for lung resection. Carbon dioxide retention and hypoxaemia are a particular risk in this group. The bicarbonate value in a preoperative arterial blood gas sample will provide a guide to the $PaCO_2$ to be expected in these patients.

Acute lung injury and postpneumonectomy pulmonary oedema

Acute respiratory distress syndrome has an overall incidence of 4% to 5% following lung resection and has been called postpneumonectomy pulmonary oedema (PPE). The term PPE also includes lobectomy patients.

Possible causes of, and contributing factors to, PPE are shown in Table 12.4.

Fluid overload has been incriminated as a cause of PPE. It is therefore recommended that fluid overload is avoided perioperatively and that a positive fluid balance should not exceed 20 ml/kg for the first 24 h (including the operative period).

Hyperinflation of the lung during one-lung ventilation (OLV) has also been incriminated as a factor contributing to PPE. Tidal volumes of 10 ml/kg during OLV approach the levels that can cause volutrauma.

Table 12.4   Factors contributing to post-pneumonectomy pulmonary oedema

- Fluid overload
- Damage to lymphatic drainage (surgical)
- Hyperinflation of lung intraoperatively ('volutrauma')
- Right ventricular dysfunction
- Reperfusion injury
- Cytokine release
- Oxygen toxicity

This is particularly so after right pneumonectomy where damage to the left lung lymphatic drainage may occur. The use of lower tidal volumes in patients with high inflation pressure or abnormal pressure–volume loops may limit ventilatory damage intraoperatively. Right ventricular dysfunction, caused by an increased afterload as the cardiac output is channelled through a smaller pulmonary vascular bed, is common following thoracotomy. An increase in right ventricular pressure in the early postoperative period often coincides with the withdrawal of supplementary oxygen. Hypercarbia contributes to an increase in pulmonary artery pressure. In high-risk patients, oxygen therapy should be continued until satisfactory saturations are sustained continuously on room air. If overt right ventricular failure is suspected clinically, and confirmed by central venous pressure measurements and echocardiography, then inotropic and pulmonary vasodilator therapy is necessary.

Cardiovascular complications and management
Hypotension
As the patient is fully rewarmed and analgesia is established, peripheral vasodilation occurs and hypotension may result. A fluid regimen of dextrose/saline solution 1 ml/kg/h (with potassium supplementation) is inadequate at this time; transfusion of colloid is required. It may be necessary to transfuse 1 l or more of colloid but, above this amount, a careful reappraisal of the patient's clinical status is required to avoid overtransfusion. If hypotension persists, despite adequate volume replacement, and blood loss into the drains is not excessive, hidden blood loss should be sought. Considerable amounts of blood can accumulate in a pneumonectomy space. A chest X-ray showing a rapidly filling space indicates that active blood loss is continuing with, or without, a drain. If hypotension persists despite adequate filling, it may be necessary to initiate inotropic therapy. A urinary catheter should also be inserted at this stage if one is not already in place.

Hypertension and myocardial ischaemia
Thoracic surgical patients often have concomitant cardiovascular disease. Anti-anginal therapy and treatment of hypertension is always continued up to and including the day of surgery and should be recommenced postoperatively. Perioperative beta blockade is likely to reduce cardiac morbidity in non-cardiac surgery. In the immediate postoperative period, hypertension can occur, particularly if analgesia is suboptimal and the patient is hypercarbic. Intravenous glyceryl trinitrate is used to control hypertension, whilst analgesia is established.

Acute blood loss

The level of acceptable blood loss, as measured by chest drainage, varies depending on the surgery. The blood loss during the first hour may be spuriously high as blood and fluid, which has collected during closure, empties through the drains, aided by the change from a supine to an upright sitting position. A subsequent blood loss of 2 ml/kg/h is cause for concern after a routine thoracotomy. If this bleeding continues for over 3 h, and a clotting screen is normal, then re-exploration is warranted, although any clotting defect should be rectified. After an operation involving an extensive surgical dissection (e.g. extrapleural pneumonectomy for a lung destroyed by chronic infection), this level of bleeding is usually tolerated over a period of 6–12 h with appropriate transfusion of blood and clotting factors. If blood loss persists postoperatively, frequent chest X-rays are necessary to ensure that blood is not sequestrating within the chest and that blood loss is not underestimated. Significant blood clot within the pleural space is an indication for re-exploration, even if visible blood losses are acceptable. A chronic haemothorax leads to a complicated postoperative course with frequent arrhythmias, episodic hypotension and a potential site for infection at a later stage.

Volume requirements may be underestimated in patients with a large amount of blood clot within the chest. Induction of anaesthesia for re-exploration and a change to the lateral position further compromises venous return and cardiac output and can result in profound hypotension. Further transfusion or even temporary vasoconstrictor therapy may be necessary.

Arrhythmias

Supraventricular arrhythmias, particularly atrial fibrillation, are common following thoracic surgery. These occur more frequently in the elderly and after pneumonectomy, particularly if there has been intrapericardial dissection. The onset is usually delayed until 2–5 days postoperatively. If indicated, digoxin is given intravenously during surgery, after checking and correcting serum potassium levels, and digitalization completed postoperatively. The onset of atrial fibrillation may be prevented, and the venticular rate will be controlled, should atrial fibrillation still occur.

If prophylaxis is not used, and atrial fibrillation occurs postoperatively, then rapid intravenous digitalization can bring the heart rate under control within a few hours. Beta adrenergic blockade is an alternative to digoxin therapy, particularly in the hypertensive patient already receiving this medication. Occasionally, direct current conversion is indicated to re-establish sinus rhythm promptly, particularly if the patient is haemodynamically unstable.

Significant ventricular dysrhythmias are treated conventionally with lidocaine or amiodarone once obvious aetiological factors such as hypoxaemia and hypokalaemia have been corrected.

Postoperative analgesia

Adequate analgesia is essential following thoracotomy, to relieve distress, improve lung function, allow effective physiotherapy and early mobilization, and reduce the incidence of postoperative complications. Pain arises from a number of sources. These include the chest wall and most of the pleura via the intercostal nerves, the diaphragmatic pleura via the phrenic nerves, the mediastinal pleura via the vagus nerve and the shoulder joint by the spinal nerves (C5–C7). Regional analgesic techniques are in widespread use following thoracic surgery (Table 12.5).

Choice of analgesic technique

Patients scheduled for lung resection and oesophageal surgery are encouraged to accept epidural analgesia. Those undergoing lesser procedures, such as video-assisted thoracoscopic surgery, are usually managed with intravenous opioids unless their operation is likely to be particularly painful (e.g. pleurectomy). Patients who decline epidural analgesia and those in whom epidural block is contraindicated, or difficult to establish, can be managed with other local analgesic techniques, such as intra- and extrapleural block (see below), combined in most cases with intravenous opioids.

Table 12.5   Regional analgesic techniques for thoracic surgery

- **Nerve blocks**
  Intercostal
  Intrapleural (intercostals)
  Extrapleural (intercostals)
  Paravertebral

- **Epidural**
  Thoracic epidural
  Lumbar epidural

Patients managed with intravenous opioids, without a local block, may require supplementation of their analgesia with non-steroidal anti-inflammatory drugs (NSAIDs) or alpha-2 adrenoreceptor agonists.

Intravenous opioids
Morphine is the major opioid used postoperatively. It is administered by a patient-controlled analgesia device or as a continuous infusion, at a rate controlled by the nursing staff. Intravenous anti-emetic therapy is given on a regular basis. Opioid analgesia has well known and significant side effects, including respiratory depression and nausea.

Supplementation of intravenous opioid analgesia
NSAIDs are often very helpful in establishing good pain relief post-thoracotomy if analgesia is inadequate with intravenous opioids: diclofenac (50–100 mg) rectally, or ketorolac (10–15 mg) intramusculary or intravenously.

The combination of NSAIDs with opioids can be extremely effective but there is a risk of renal failure and exacerbation of postoperative bleeding. NSAIDs are only given to patients with normal renal function.

Local anaesthetic techniques
Intercostal/intrapleural/extrapleural block
The intercostal nerves can be blocked by a simple 'one-shot' injection technique, or more commonly via a catheter placed between the visceral and parietal pleurae (intra- or interpleural method), or by way of a catheter placed in an extrapleural pocket.

Simple intercostal blocks can be performed by the surgeon before chest closure. They ameliorate wound and drain site pain initially, but are short-lived and do not influence extensive chest wall pain.

Intrapleural catheters can be sited by the anaesthetist or surgeon between the visceral and parietal pleura where the spread of local anaesthetic agent is not contained. Other major drawbacks to this technique are that large volumes of local anaesthetic agent are lost through the chest drains and high plasma levels of agent occur, with the risk of toxicity.

Extrapleural catheters are placed by the surgeon at the end of surgery and tunnelled out of the chest via a Tuohy needle. Local anaesthetic agents are then infused down the catheter into the prepared pocket.

Paravetebral block

Paravetebral block can be performed as a single-shot technique or with the insertion of a catheter. Multiple intercostal nerves can be blocked by a single paravertebral injection. The block produces good analgesia with the advantage of unilateral sympathetic blockade, and therefore a lesser degree of hypotension than with a thoracic epidural. Paravertebral block is easier to perform than a thoracic epidural, but the quality of pain relief is inferior.

Epidural analgesia

Thoracic epidural analgesia is the preferred analgesic technique in high-risk patients. The combination of a low dose local anaesthetic agent (bupivacaine 0.1%) with a lipophilic opioid, such as fentanyl, provides good analgesia without the profound sympathetic blockade associated with higher doses of local anaesthetic. Apart from possible hypotension and bradycardia caused by local anaesthetic agents, epidural opioids can result in respiratory depression, nausea, pruritus and urinary retention. Patients should therefore be nursed in an HDU.

The question of anticoagulation and epidural placement must be considered. Preoperative low-molecular-weight heparin is omitted in patients likely to have epidural analgesia and the catheter removed approximately 2 h before another a dose of heparin is due in the postoperative period.

Miscellaneous management problems

Thromboprophylaxis

Antithrombosis prophylaxis is undertaken in all patients, except young 'fit' patients having short operations. Antithromboembolism stockings, however, are prescribed, in all groups. Patients are classified as moderate or high risk of developing postoperative venous thromboembolism, and are treated accordingly.

Moderate-risk patients are all those having major surgery together with debilitated patients having any type of operation. High-risk patients include those with malignancy, a previous history of deep vein thrombosis, the morbidly obese and those aged over 65 years. Patients who have recently undertaken a long-haul flight must also be considered high-risk as should women using oral contraceptives. The contraceptive pill is discontinued 1 month prior to surgery, but hormone replacement therapy is continued.

Moderate- and high-risk patients are nursed with stockings and given low-molecular-weight heparin perioperatively by once daily subcutaneous injection. Standard prophylactic regimens do not require monitoring.

Antibiotic prophylaxis
Antibiotic prophylaxis should be kept simple. The majority of patients are given a first generation cephalosporin, such as cephazolin, during, or just after, the induction of anaesthesia and continued for 24 h postoperatively. Antibiotic prophylaxis is particularly important if surgery involves the opening of the trachea, bronchus or oesophagus, or if the patient is immunosuppressed. Metronidazole is given in addition to cephazolin in all patients undergoing tracheal resection, oesophagectomy and excision of abdominal metastases.

If a thoracotomy is undertaken in the presence of an obstructed airway or pleural sepsis, or prosthetic material is introduced (chest wall prosthesis, vascular graft), broader spectrum cover is used with the addition of teicoplanin and metronidazole to the cephalosporin regime.

Renal failure
Causative factors include pre-existing renal dysfunction, dehydration, cardiovascular complications and the use of nephrotoxic drugs, such as aminoglycoside antibiotics and NSAIDs.

Urinary retention is common following thoracotomy, particularly in elderly male patients and those with epidural analgesia. If there is any doubt about the urine output, a urinary catheter should be inserted. A urine output > 0.5 ml/kg/h must be maintained in the immediate postoperative period. It is important to exclude, and treat, hypovolaemia before using a diuretic such as frusemide to promote urine output.

Nutrition
Patients presenting for lung resection are rarely grossly cachetic or malnourished. Following thoracotomy, patients should be encouraged to supplement their oral diet with liquid calorie and protein supplements. Occasionally, it is necessary to insert a fine bore nasogastric tube to provide a route for enteral feeding. These are uncomfortable and interfere with coughing and sputum clearance.

Patients with oesophageal obstruction may be grossly malnourished and need enteral feeding preoperatively, either through a fine bore nasogastric tube inserted through the obstruction, or via a percutaneous endoscopic gastrostomy feeding tube.

Further reading

Azad SC. Perioperative pain management in patients undergoing thoracic surgery. Curr Opin Anaesthesiol 2001;14:87–91.

Bardoczky GI, Levarlet M, Engelman E, Defrancquen P. Continuous spirometry for detection of double-lumen endobrochial tube displacement. Br J Anaesth 1993;70:499–502.

Bromage PR. The control of post-thoracotomy pain. Anaesthesia 1989;44: 445–446.

Cina RA, Froehlich JB, Hamdan AD. Perioperative β-blockade to reduce cardiac morbidity in noncardiac surgery. In: Park KW (ed.). Preoperative cardiac evaluation. International anesthesiology clinics, vol. 39; Philadelphia: Lippincott Williams & Wilkins; 2001. pp. 93–104.

Entwistle MD, Roe PG, Sapsford DJ, Berrisford RG, Jones JG. Patterns of oxygenation after thoracotomy. Br J Anaesth 1991;67:704–711.

Goldstraw P. Postoperative management of the thoracic surgical patient. In: Gothard JWW (ed.). Thoracic anaesthesia. Clinical anaesthesiology, vol. 1. London: Baillière Tindall; 1987. pp. 207–231.

Hardy I, Ahmed S. Pain control following thoracic surgery. In: Gosh S, Latimer RD (eds). Thoracic anaesthesia. Principles and practice. Oxford: Butterworth Heinemann; 1999.

Horlocker TT, Wedel DJ. Spinal and epidural blockade and perioperative low molecular weight heparin: smooth sailing on the Titanic. Anesth Analg 1998;86:1153–1156.

Kam AC, O'Brien M, Kam PCA. Pleural drainage systems. Anaesthesia 1993; 48.154–161.

Maze M, Tranquill W. Alpha-2 adrenoreceptor agonists. Defining the role in clinical anesthesia. Anesthesiology 1991;74:581–605.

Simon BA, Hurford WE, Alfille PH, Haspel K, Behringer EC. An aid in the diagnosis of malpositioned double-lumen tubes. Anesthesiology 1992;76: 845.

Slinger PD. Perioperative fluid management for thoracic surgery: the puzzle of postpneumonectomy pulmonary edema. J Cardiothorac Vasc Anesth 1995; 9:442–451.

Vaughan RS. Pain relief after thoracotomy (editorial). Br J Anaesth 2001; 87:681–683.

Index